BRAGG

APPLE CIDER VINEGAR

VINEGAR

MIRACLE HEALTH SYSTEM

with the

BRAGG HEALTHY LIFESTYLE

Blueprint for Physical, Mental and Spiritual Improvement – Healthy, Vital Living to 120

Genesis 6:3

PAUL C. BRAGG, N.D., Ph.D.
LIFE EXTENSION SPECIALIST

and

PATRICIA BRAGG, N.D., Ph.D.
HEALTH & FITNESS EXPERT

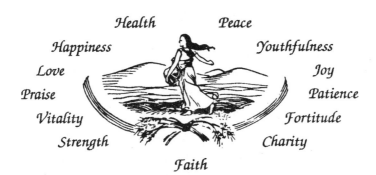

Health   Peace

Happiness   Youthfulness

Love   Joy

Praise   Patience

Vitality   Fortitude

Strength   Charity

Faith

JOIN
Bragg Health Crusades for a 100% Healthy World for All!

HEALTH SCIENCE
Box 7, Santa Barbara, California 93102 USA

World Wide Web: www.bragg.com

BRAGG
APPLE CIDER
VINEGAR

MIRACLE HEALTH SYSTEM

PAUL C. BRAGG, N.D., Ph.D.
LIFE EXTENSION SPECIALIST
and
PATRICIA BRAGG, N.D., Ph.D.
HEALTH & FITNESS EXPERT

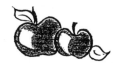

**To see Bragg Books and products on-line, visit our World Wide Web Site at: www.bragg.com
e-mail address: bragg@bragg.com**

Quantity Purchases: Companies, Professional Groups, Churches, Clubs, Fundraisers etc. Please contact our Special Sales Department.

♻ This book is printed on recycled, acid-free paper.

- REVISED AND EXPANDED -
Copyright © Health Science

FiftyFirst printing MCMXCVIX
ISBN: 0-87790-042-6

Published in the United States
HEALTH SCIENCE, Box 7, Santa Barbara, California 93102 USA

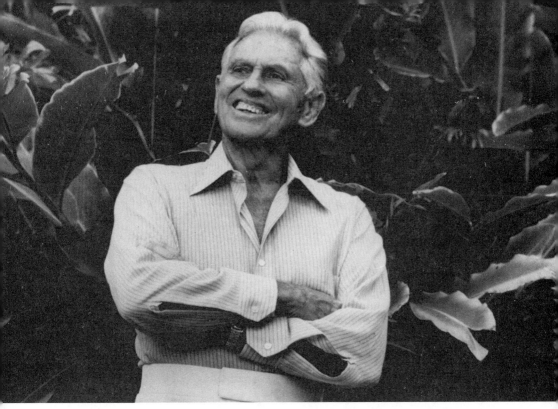

PAUL C. BRAGG, N.D., Ph.D.
World's Leading Healthy Lifestyle Authority

Paul C. Bragg's daughter Patricia and their wonderful, healthy members of the Bragg *Longer Life, Health and Happiness Club* exercise daily on the beautiful Fort DeRussy lawn, at world famous Waikiki Beach in Honolulu, Hawaii. Membership is free and open to everyone who wishes to attend any morning – Monday through Saturday, from 9 to 10:30 am – for Bragg Deep Breathing and health and fitness exercises. On Saturday there are often health lectures on how to live a long, healthy life! The group averages 75 to 125 per day, depending on the season. From December to March it can go up to 200. Its dedicated leaders have been carrying on the class for over 27 years. Thousands have visited the club from around the world and carried the Bragg health and fitness message to friends and relatives back home. When you visit Honolulu, Hawaii, Patricia invites you and your friends to join her and the club for wholesome, healthy fellowship. She also recommends you visit the outer Hawaiian Islands (Kauai, Hawaii, Maui, Molokai) for a fulfilling, healthy vacation.

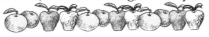

iii

To maintain good health, normal weight and increase the good life of radiant health, joy and happiness, the body must be exercised properly (stretching, walking, jogging, running, biking, swimming, deep breathing, good posture, etc.) and nourished wisely with natural foods. – Paul C. Bragg

KEEP HEALTHY & YOUTHFUL BIOLOGICALLY WITH EXERCISE & GOOD NUTRITION

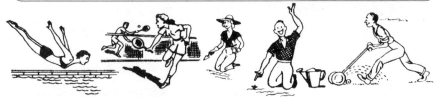

Always remember you have the following important reasons for following The Bragg Healthy Lifestyle:

- The ironclad laws of Mother Nature and God.
- Your common sense, which tells you that you are doing right.
- Your aim to make your health better and your life longer.
- Your resolve to prevent illness so that you may enjoy life.
- Make an art of healthy living; you will be youthful at any age.
- You will retain your faculties and be hale, hearty, active and useful far beyond the ordinary length of years.
- You will also possess superior mental and physical powers!

WANTED – For Robbing Health & Life

KILLER Saturated Fats

CLOGGER Salt

DOPEY Caffeine

PLUGGER Frying Pan

DEATH-DEALER Drugs

GREASY Overweight

HOGGY Overeating

CHOKER Hydrogenated Fats

DEADEYED Devitalized Foods

HARD WATER Inorganic Minerals

JERKY Turbulent Emotions

CRAZY Alcohol

SMOKY Tobacco

LOAFER Laziness

What Wise Men Say

Wisdom does not show itself so much in precept as in life – a firmness of mind and mastery of appetite. – Seneca

Govern well thy appetite, lest Sin surprise thee, & her black attendant, Death. – Milton

Our prayers should be for a sound mind in a healthy body. – Juvenal

I saw few die of hunger – of eating, a hundred thousand. – Ben Franklin

Health consists of temperance alone. – Pope

Health is...a blessing that money cannot buy. – Izaak Walton

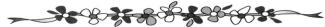

The natural healing force within us is the greatest force in getting well. – Hippocrates, Father of Medicine

iv

Of all the knowledge, that most worth having is the knowledge about health! The first requisite of a good life is to be a healthy person. – Herbert Spencer

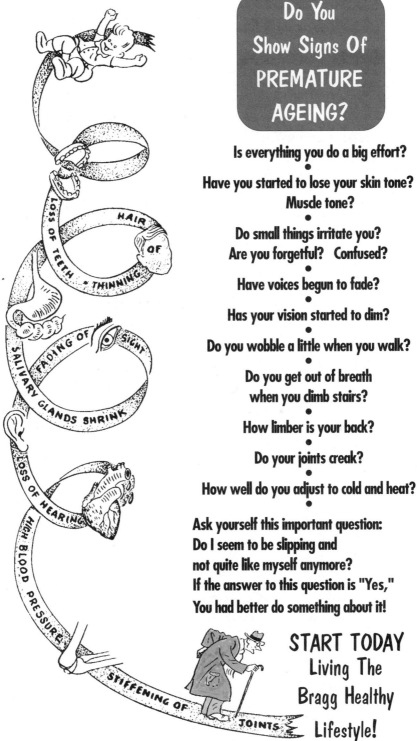

Do You Show Signs Of PREMATURE AGEING?

Is everything you do a big effort?

Have you started to lose your skin tone?
Muscle tone?

Do small things irritate you?
Are you forgetful?   Confused?

Have voices begun to fade?

Has your vision started to dim?

Do you wobble a little when you walk?

Do you get out of breath
when you climb stairs?

How limber is your back?

Do your joints creak?

How well do you adjust to cold and heat?

Ask yourself this important question:
Do I seem to be slipping and
not quite like myself anymore?
If the answer to this question is "Yes,"
You had better do something about it!

START TODAY Living The Bragg Healthy Lifestyle!

v

He who understands nature walks with God. – Edgar Cayce

BRAGG HEALTH CRUSADES for the 21st CENTURY
Teaching People Worldwide to Live
Healthier, Stronger Lives for a Better World

We love sharing, teaching and giving, and you can share this love by being a partner with Bragg Health Crusades Worldwide Outreach. Bragg Crusades is dedicated to helping others! We feel blessed when your life improves through following our teachings from the Bragg Books and Crusades. It makes all our years of faithful service so worthwhile!

The Miracle of Fasting book has been the #1 book for 13 years in Russia! Why? Because we show them how to live a healthy, wholesome life for less money, and it's so easy to understand and follow. Most healthful lifestyle habits are free (eg. - good posture, clean thoughts, plain natural foods, exercise and deep breathing, that draws energy into the body). We continue to reach the multitudes with all our health teachings, lectures, Crusades, radio, TV and video outreaches.

My joy and priorities come from God and healthy living. I'm excited about spreading health worldwide, for now it's needed more than ever! My father and I also pioneered Health TV with our program "Health and Happiness" filmed in Hollywood. It's thrilling to be a Health Crusader and you will enjoy it also. See back pages to list names (yourself, family, friends) who you think would like to receive our free Health Bulletins!

By reading Bragg Self-Health Books you gain a new confidence that you can help yourself, family and friends to Healthy Principles of Living! Please call your local health store and book store and ask for the Bragg Health Books. Prayerfully, we hope to have all stores stock the Bragg Books so they will be available to everyone.

I have visions of **Health Retreats** where people can find joyous health and rebirth! They will be **Recharging - Physically, Mentally, Emotionally and Spiritually**. Everyone needs retreats now, more than ever!

For the new millennium, we are planning Bragg Recharge Retreats and Child & Senior Care Centers which are desperately needed across America. We are just waiting for the right locations and funding. We can accept all gifts, monetary and land (appraised value), and we can give a receipt for tax deductions. Seldom-used ranches, farms and old estates could become Recharge Centers for rejuvenating mind, body and soul. Those attending would become health crusaders for their families and friends. Empty buildings and spacious older homes with yards would make ideal Child & Senior Centers. If you have a location and would like to be part of this great outreach, please call or write to me.

We are not new to retreats; I was reared on retreats. Holidays and vacations were spent at camp and retreats for precious weeks of growth and recharge. My Dad pioneered the first health spa (Macfadden's Deauville) in Miami Beach and others in Highland Springs, CA, and Danville, NY.

I expend all my energy and funds inspiring and helping others to help and heal themselves! Genuine love seeks ways to express itself! I thank you for your caring, sharing support – with your help we can achieve our future goals! I know God will bless you. Your needed help will be a blessing to The Bragg Health Crusades. Our budget is for a mighty worthwhile cause. I know you, your family and friends will enjoy and benefit from our teachings and health retreats.

With A Loving, Grateful Heart, *Patricia Bragg*

BRAGG HEALTH CRUSADES, America's Health Pioneers

A non-profit organization. Gifts are tax deductible.
7340 Hollister Ave., Santa Barbara, CA 93117 USA (805) 968-1020

Over 85 continuous years spreading health & fitness worldwide

Contents

In 400 B.C., Hippocrates, the Father of Medicine, treated his patients with amazing raw Apple Cider Vinegar because he recognized its powerful cleansing and healing qualities. It's a naturally occurring antibiotic and antiseptic that fights germs and bacteria.

Title

*"Open thou thine eyes, that I may behold
wondrous things out of thy law."* – Psalms 119:18

Astronomers Find Vinegar in Distant Space

*In a stellar cloud 25,000 light years from Earth, researchers
recently found organic vinegar, a molecule that may have played
a big role in the formation of life.* – University of Chicago

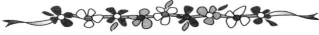

Contents

*When you sell a man a book you don't just sell him paper, ink and glue,
you sell him a whole new life! There's heaven and earth in a real book.
The real purpose of books is to inspire the mind to do its own thinking!*
– Christopher Morely

Contents

Bragg Healthy Lifestyle Plan

- *Read, plan, plot and follow through for supreme health and longevity.*
- *Organizing your lifestyle helps you identify what's important in your life.*
- *Where space allows we have included "words of wisdom" from*
  great minds to motivate and inspire you.
- *Underline, highlight or dog-ear pages as you read important passages.*
- *Be faithful to your health goals everyday for a healthy, strong, happy life.*

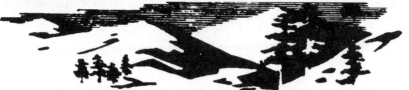

TEN HEALTH COMMANDMENTS

Thou shall respect and protect thy body as the
highest manifestation of life.

Thou shall abstain from all unnatural, devitalized
food and stimulating beverages.

Thou shall nourish thy body with only Natural
unprocessed, live foods, that . . .

Thou shall extend thy years in health for loving,
sharing with others and charitable service.

Thou shall regenerate thy body by the right balance
of activity and rest.

Thou shall purify thy cells, tissues and blood with
healthy foods, pure water, fresh air and sunshine.

Thou shall abstain from all food when out of sorts
in mind or body.

Thou shall keep all thoughts, words and emotions
pure, good, calm, kind, uplifting and loving.

Thou shall increase thy knowledge of Nature's Laws,
follow them and enjoy the fruits of thy life's labor.

Thou shall lift up thyself, friends and family by
obedience to God's Healthy, Pure Laws of Living.

Paul C. Bragg   *Patricia Bragg*

Morning Resolve

I will this day live a simple, sincere and serene life, repelling
promptly every thought of impurity, discontent, anxiety, anger
discouragement and self-seeking. I will cultivate cheerfulness,
happiness, charity and the love of brotherhood; exercising economy
in expenditure, generosity in giving, carefulness in conversation and
diligence in appointed service. I pledge fidelity to every trust and a
childlike faith in God, in particular, I will be faithful in those habits of
prayer, study, work, physical exercise, deep breathing and good posture.
I shall fast one 24 hour period each week, eat only natural foods and
get sufficient sleep each night. I will make every effort to improve myself
physically, mentally, emotionally and spiritually every day.

Morning Prayer used by Paul C. Bragg and Patricia Bragg

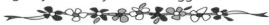

*Wake up and say, "Today I am going to be happier, healthier and wiser
in my daily living as I am the captain of my life and am going to steer it
for 100% healthy lifestyle living!". . . Fact: Happy people look younger,
live longer, happier and have fewer health problems!* – Patricia Bragg

Bragg
Apple Cider Vinegar
Miracle Health System

How to Use The
Powerful Health Qualities
of Natural Apple Cider Vinegar

Research worldwide supports and commends what Hippocrates (the father of medicine) found and treated his patients with in 400 B.C. He discovered that natural, undistilled Apple Cider Vinegar (or ACV)* is a powerful cleansing and healing elixir – a naturally occurring antibiotic and antiseptic that fights germs and bacteria – for a healthier, stronger, longer life!

The versatility of ACV as a powerful body cleansing agent is legendary. It's been traced to Egyptian urns as far back as 3000 B.C. The Babylonians used it as a condiment and preservative, while Julius Caesar's army used ACV tonic to stay healthy and fight off disease. The Greeks and Romans kept vinegar vessels for healing and flavoring. It was used in Biblical times as an antiseptic and a healing agent and is mentioned in the Bible. In Paris in the Middle Ages it was sold from barrels by street vendors as a body deodorant, healing tonic and a health vinegar drink.

1

Even Christopher Columbus and his crew on his voyage to discover America in 1492 had their vinegar barrels for prevention of scurvy as did the soldiers in the American Civil War. For centuries in Japan, the feared Samurai warriors drank it for strength and power. ACV has been used for thousands of years not only for health reasons, but also as a cleansing agent to remove bacteria, germs, odors, and even stains and spots.

A teacher for the day can be a guiding light for a lifetime!
Bragg books are silent health teachers - never tiring, ready night or day to help you help yourself to health! Our books are written with love and a deep desire to guide you to a healthy lifestyle. – Patricia Bragg

*The best is the organic, raw, unfiltered, unpasteurized apple cider vinegar with the "mother," available most Health Stores. See back pages for info.

ACV – Mother Nature's Perfect Food

Natural (undistilled) organic, raw ACV can really be called one of Mother Nature's most perfect foods. It is made from fresh, crushed apples which are then allowed to mature naturally in wooden barrels, as wood seems to "boost" the natural fermentation. Natural ACV should be a rich, brownish color and if held to the light you might see a tiny formation of "cobweb-like" substances that we call the "mother." Usually some "mother" will show in the bottom of the ACV bottle the more it ages. It never needs refrigeration. You can also save some "mother" and transfer it to work in other natural vinegars. When you smell natural ACV, there's a pungent odor and sometimes it's so ripened it puckers your mouth and smarts your eyes – these are natural, good signs.

Why Has Natural Apple Cider Vinegar Disappeared from Grocers' Shelves?

The blame for the disappearance of natural raw apple cider vinegar from supermarkets lies on the shoulders of the general public, as well as the producers of vinegar.

Most people buy food with their eyes, not thinking of good nutrition. The vinegar producers failed to enlighten the public on what powerful health qualities were locked within natural ACV. Why? Because most of them had not the slightest knowledge of the health values of natural, raw, organic, unfiltered, cloudy (and to some, less attractive-looking) apple cider vinegar with the "mother." They produced pasteurized, refined and distilled vinegars because the public demanded the clear look. It was simply filling current supply and demand.

Powerful Health Qualities Removed

You cannot completely blame the producers of vinegar. They are not nutritionists, nor are they biochemists. Their business is to give the customers what they want. Most people purchase vinegar for flavoring, also for pickling and marinating their foods. Some women use it to rinse their hair after shampooing, as it leaves it squeaky clean, softer and much easier to manage.

ACV is also a great germ fighter in the home, lab, etc.. Some mix it with water to wash windows, as it removes sludge and keeps them sparkling clean. ACV has hundreds of uses and its versatility is legendary as a powerful household cleansing and deodorizing agent free of dangerous chemicals. (See pages 102 to 104 for vinegar cleaning hints.)

ACV Has Powerful Health Qualities

Both the general public and the producers of vinegar have been uninformed as to the powerful health qualities of organic, raw, unfiltered, fully ripened ACV. Ignorance isn't always bliss! When most people see natural apple cider vinegar with the brownish color and the tiny, cobweb "mother" floating in it, they think it looks unappetizing. The general public has been educated and brainwashed to want everything they purchase to have perfect eye appeal!

To meet this demand that vinegar must be clear and light colored and free from the brownish, cobweb "mother" is the reason producers distill their vinegar. In distilling, the vinegar is turned to steam by heating. Therefore it destroys the powerful enzymes and distills out the life-giving minerals such as potassium, phosphorus, natural organic sodium, magnesium, sulphur, iron, copper, natural organic fluorine, silicon, trace minerals and pectin and many other powerful nutrients! Distilling also destroys the natural malic and tartaric acids which are important in fighting body toxins and inhibiting unfriendly bacteria.

You can see how the public, with their obsession for *eye appeal foods,* reacts. The producers of apple cider vinegar, who agreed to sell their product for a profit, put a "death warrant" against healthy, organic, raw, fully ripened ACV. The public got what they wanted – a clear, appealing, but dead ACV. When natural ACV was hard to find, other strange vinegars began to appear on grocery shelves. The first was malt vinegar, a refined vinegar. It's clear and acceptable to the public. It tastes like vinegar, but has none of the healing qualities of natural, raw ACV.

The universally accepted #1 fruit, the apple, is popular across America and around the world. Early American settlers, the Pilgrims, brought apples to America in the 1600s and became Johnny Appleseeders, starting apple orchards that eventually spread throughout America.

Commercial Vinegars are Real Tragedies

Then came the real tragedy: a food chemist produced an imitation vinegar from coal tar! It looked clean, white and tasted like vinegar. Today it's the most popular vinegar in supermarkets. It's cheaper than distilled vinegar or malt vinegar. Most people buy these worthless vinegars. There's nothing good about commercial vinegars, except they look clean and taste like vinegar. They have no health value! They don't contain the health values of organic, raw ACV with the *mother*. Millions worldwide never get the health benefits of this natural ACV as Hippocrates used in 400 B.C.

Millions Suffer from Malnutrition

"Mal" means bad. As a consequence of not getting natural, healthy, balanced diets, millions worldwide suffer from many forms of subclinical malnutrition. This means many people, due to vitamin and mineral deficiencies, feel half-sick most of the time! They lack vim, vigor and "Go Power" and feel tired most of the time. Their daily food intake and the commercial vinegars they use don't provide sufficient vitamins and minerals, nor the potassium their bodies require. They lack vital power and feel exhausted. This is the reason people turn to stimulants like coffee, America's most popular unhealthy drink, and to colas, alcohol, cigarettes and over-the-counter "fix-all" drugs. After these stimulants' effects wear off, they feel terrible. They just exist, and are not living happy, healthy lives!

Coffee – America's #1 Drug Addiction

Coffee drinking (caffeine) is the #1 drug addiction in America! Millions of pounds of coffee are sold to America yearly. That's not to mention the caffeine in soft drinks. Plus there's millions of addicted chocoholics who are hooked on chocolate and sugar – a harmful combination. The shocking list of caffeine-related side effects include: high blood pressure, hypertension, arrythmia, elevated cholesterol, glucose, increased tendencies to allergies, chronic fatigue and autoimmune disorders, etc.

Man is fully responsible for his nature and his choices. – Jean-Paul Sartre

You see these unhappy people about you every day. They are washed out and ageing prematurely. Many lack skin and muscle tone and have dark circles and puffy (water) bags under their eyes. Their eyes lose the sparkle of health and youthfulness and become like dead fish eyes. Malnourished people are mostly lifeless and everything they do requires a tremendous effort. They are not really living and most are not happy. Many suffer from depression and mental fatigue – nerve burnout.

Apples Are Rich in Potassium & Enzymes

"An apple a day keeps the doctor away" is a familiar saying to millions. It carries good common sense. The apple is one of God's great health-giving foods.

Apples are a rich source of potassium, which is to the soft tissues of the body as calcium is to the bones and harder tissues. Potassium is the mineral of youthfulness; it is the "artery softener," keeping the arteries of the body flexible and resilient. It is a fighter of dangerous bacteria and viruses. Yes, when you say, "An apple a day keeps the doctor away," you are talking good, down-to-earth old-fashioned folk medicine for vibrant health!

The apple has stood the test of time. It is one of the oldest known fruits that humans consume. Since the Garden of Eden the apple has played a vital part in our destiny. People have been eating apples for thousands of years. Apple eaters have a certain healthfulness that non-apple eaters never achieve.

Apples are delicious fruits that most people enjoy eating, but we look on the apple as more than something good to eat. Potassium is the key mineral in the constellation of minerals; it's so important to every living thing that without it there would be no life!

Most humans are deficient in potassium and it reflects in their cell tissues and throughout their entire body. Look around you. How many people do you see that have the super glow of health?

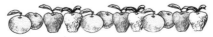

There is no wealth greater than the health of the body. – The Bible

Millions Suffer From Potassium Deficiency

Millions living in today's civilization and eating its commercialized, processed foods have a potassium deficiency. The skin and muscle tone are bad. The flesh does not cling firmly to the body's bony framework. Lines and wrinkles fill the face and neck.

One sign is flabby, excess skin hanging over the eyes. If the potassium deficiency continues, the prolapsing eyelids progress. Soon, people are looking out of little slits instead of wide-open eyes. Thousands have turned to eyelid surgery to correct droopy eyelids, also called hooded eyelids, that roll down and rest on their eyelashes causing eyestrain, headaches, etc. If an eye doctor suggests corrective surgery for this, the insurance company usually honors the claim. It's an in/out local procedure. It's best the eye surgeon is board certified. People wrongly blame droopy eyes, physical changes in the skin and lack of muscle tone on their age.

But the truth is . . . you must have potassium to build and maintain youthful, healthy tissues! If you do not get your required amount of potassium daily, you soon acquire an old-age look. This is premature ageing due to potassium deficiency and unhealthy living!

It is the same in your flower and vegetable garden. Potassium is necessary for the production of the substances that give rigidity to plant stems and increase their resistance to the many diseases that attack plants. Potassium is also the powerful element that changes seeds into plants and beautiful flowers by progressive development. If plants become deficient in potassium, they stop their growth. If the potassium deficiency is not corrected, the plant slowly starts to wither, turns yellow and dies! The same is true of animals and humans with a potassium deficiency: there is a slow degeneration leading to death of the cells, then death of life.

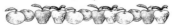

Every day the average heart, your best friend, beats 100,000 times and pumps 2,000 gallons of blood for nourishing your body. In about 70 years that adds up to more than 360 million (faithful) heartbeats. Please be good to your heart and live The Bragg Healthy Lifestyle for a long, happy, healthy life! Here's to Genesis 6:3 for you. –Patricia Bragg

Refined Foods & Flours Remove Vital Potassium which Causes Poor Health!

Robbed grains: The miller refines and processes our grains to get white flour that will keep for years . . . that becomes the staff of death! Even bugs have more sense – they won't eat it because it has been robbed of its potassium and vital life-giving qualities!

Shocking loss of potassium and nutrients in making white flour: In milling wheat, the miller refines out 25 important food elements, including vital amino acids, vitamin E, bran, the rich B-complex vitamins and potassium. Cows fed refined grain, with the potassium milled out and de-germed, die early of heart failure.

The more they refine vital potassium out of foods, the sicker Americans get: People waste money, time, and energy and suffer the loss of health by being sick. The #1 health plan should be to teach Americans how to live a healthy lifestyle that maintains health by correct eating and living habits. Healthy nutrition will create bones that last a lifetime, cells that resist disease and arteries that stay healthy, cholesterol-free and unclogged!

Bad Nutrition – #1 Cause of Sickness

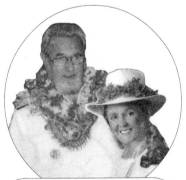

Dr. Koop & Patricia

"Diet-related diseases account for 68% of all deaths."

Dr. C. Everett Koop, our friend and America's former Surgeon General said this in his famous 1988 landmark report on nutrition and health in America. People don't die of infectious conditions as such, but of malnutrition that allows the germs to get a foothold in sickly bodies. Also, bad nutrition is usually the main cause of noninfectious, fatal or degenerative conditions. When the body has its full vitamin and mineral quota, including precious potassium, it's almost impossible for germs to get a foothold in a healthy, powerful bloodstream and tissues!

The Body Has the Seed of Eternal Life

Outside of fatal accidents, there is no reason why a person should leave before his or her time. It has been proven by some of the greatest scientific minds that there are no special diseases of old age. A person should not die simply because they live to 60, 70, 80 or 90 years of age, because calendar age is not toxic. People create their toxins by their eating and living habits.

Most people die of some fatal condition that they have built into their bodies by incorrect living or by violating the natural laws that govern the physical body.

The two great enemies of life are toxic poisons (found in food, air, water and soil) and nutritional deficiencies caused by improper diet. The best prevention of sickness is to eat vital, healthy foods (organic when possible), especially those high in potassium. These provide the body with correct, life-giving nourishment.

Every 90 days a new bloodstream, the river of life, is built in the body by the food you eat, the liquid you drink and the air you breathe. From the bloodstream the body's cells are made, nourished and maintained. Every 11 months we have a new set of billions of miraculous body cells, and every 2 years we have an entirely new set of bones and hard tissues. There is no reason to get old because the body is constantly cleansing and renewing its cells to keep your precious human temple healthy for life.

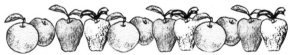

The laws of health are inexorable; we see people going down and out in their prime of life because no attention is paid to them!
– Paul C. Bragg

Age does not depend upon years, but upon temperament and health.
– Tyron Edwards

Your Daily Habits Form Your Future
Habits can be right or wrong, good or bad, healthy or unhealthy, rewarding or unrewarding. The right or wrong habits, decisions, actions, words or deeds . . . are up to you! Wisely choose your habits, as they can make or break you and your health! – Patricia Bragg

Exercise Helps Keep You More Youthful, Healthier, Stronger, Flexible and Trim

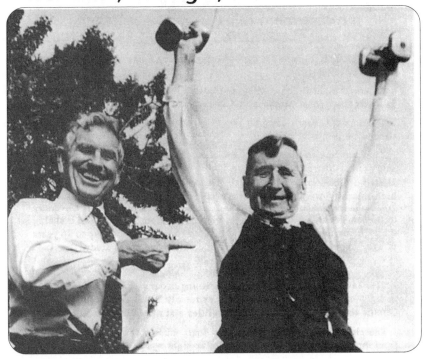

Paul C. Bragg and Friend, Roy White, 106 Years Young

Paul and Roy practiced progressive weight training 3 times a week to stay healthy and fit. Scientists have proven that weight training works miracles for all ages by maintaining more flexibility, energy and youthful stamina!

See pages 88-90 for some of the amazing scientific data coming in from around the world on the important longevity, health, renewing and rewarding benefits of regular exercise and living a healthy lifestyle!

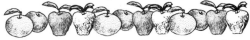

Never shatter someone else's dreams or hopes;
these are as precious, and as rare, as life itself.

Man is the sole and absolute master of his own fate forever.
What he has sown in the times of his ignorance, he must
inevitably reap; when he attains enlightenment, it is for him to
sow what he chooses and reap accordingly. – Geraldine Coster

Change your mind and change your life.

Dream big, think big, but enjoy the small miracles of everyday life!

Dr. Alexis Carrel's Great Life Extension Experiment

In his famous experiment years ago in New York, research scientist Dr. Alexis Carrel kept the cells of an embryo chicken heart alive and healthy for over 30 years by daily monitoring its complete nutrition, cleansing and elimination. A chicken's lifespan averages 7 years!

Apple cider vinegar was given to the chicken embryo daily for its full quota of potassium. Dr. Carrel definitively proved to the entire world that the body has a seed of eternal life. He could have continued this experiment indefinitely to give the embryo immortality, but felt 30 years proved the point that man kills himself by his wrong habits of overeating and living an unhealthy lifestyle. This experiment showed us the vital importance of apple cider vinegar to life, health and longevity!

Recently a remarkable study on longevity was done with earthworms. By monitoring their food intake, then decreasing it to only what was nutritionally necessary, these worms multiplied their lifespan (see bottom page 55). The results from these and many other studies have revealed the key to longer life. Many scientists know no reason why these same principles could not apply to everyone. Even today the Hunzas of Kashmir and the Georgians of Russia lead active lives to 120 and older!

Potassium Deficiency Can Stunt Growth

We have made over 10 scientific nutritional expeditions throughout the world, studying the health, longevity and growth of various races of people. We found areas where the topsoil was deficient in potassium and the people living off foods grown from this potassium-deficient soil were prone to be stunted in growth and have a shorter lifespan. The pygmies of Africa are stunted and short-lived. The same is true of the Arctic Eskimos. In their daily diet, they just do not get the required amount of potassium and other minerals that are so important to growth, health and long life.

The strongest principle of growth lies in the human choice. – George Elliot

Mentally Handicapped Children and Adults Suffer from Potassium Deficiency

We have closely studied the relationship between mentally handicapped children and adults and potassium deficiency. Many years ago, my dad brought three of these children to our home for study and observation. Three times daily – in morning, noon and night – the children had the ACV drink (1 tsp. ACV and 1 tsp. raw honey in glass of distilled water, both rich in potassium). Dad put the children on The Bragg Healthy Lifestyle which gave them extra amounts of wonderful potassium. Daily they were given multiple vitamin-mineral supplements and some niacin (50 mgs – vitamin B-3). In 3 weeks, these children became more mentally alert. After living in our home for less than a year, they were able to resume their schooling with children their own age!

Another amazing study – we brought three mentally handicapped adults into our home and after putting them on the ACV routine plus living The Bragg Healthy Lifestyle, they became self-supporting in less than a year!

Potassium Deficiency Produces Senility

Throughout the world, there are millions of senile, prematurely old people. Many of them don't know their own names, nor can they recognize their family or closest friends. They are just barely existing. It might seem that they have degenerated so much that it's almost a hopeless task to try to save them, but please always try!

We believe that many of them can be restored to useful lives if the toxic poisons are flushed from their bodies and their grave nutritional deficiencies are corrected!

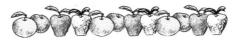

Be a Shining Star . . . *Rise above any problems – you are not locked into unhealthy habits – remember you are the captain and can guide your being into a fresh, exciting, new life filled with wonderful challenges, so get ready to take off for Super Health on Earth!* – Patricia Bragg

We choose our joys and sorrows long before we experience them. – Kahlil Gibran

Miracles with Potassium

Years ago, we selected four senile people we felt could be helped. We put them on The Bragg Healthy Lifestyle with the ACV drink and healthy foods rich in potassium. Out of the four, we were able to save three of them. All three left the convalescent home where they had been confined and became healthy, happy and self-sufficient. Two of them made remarkable recoveries. One went back to contracting and building at 83, and the other in his mid 80s resumed his accounting career!

Most senile people suffer from a clogged arterial system. Potassium is to the soft tissues of the body as calcium is to the hard structures. The potassium goes into the clogged, caked arteries and cleans out the rust and dirt just like vinegar water removes grime from windows. One can't think clearly if the arteries are heavily clogged with cholesterol and toxic poisons.

Potassium might be called the great detergent of the arteries. Potassium slows down the hardening and clogging processes that cause deadly harm to the whole cardiovascular system. Organic, raw ACV contains the miraculous potassium that makes the flesh of farm animals healthier and more tender. There is very little doubt, in animal and man, that the main function of potassium is to keep the tissues healthy, soft and pliable, and to help prevent heart attacks and strokes!

Paul Bragg Talks about Vinegar Miracles on His Family's Farm in His Youth

Long years of research have proven to me that natural apple cider vinegar is a potent source of potassium. I was raised on a large farm. On this farm, we grew many varieties of apples. I was a great apple eater. Each year my father made natural apple cider vinegar and stored it in wooden barrels. On our table we used this natural apple cider vinegar and our large family loved it.

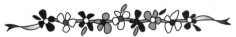

Nutrition directly affects growth, development, reproduction and well-being of an individual's physical and mental condition. Health depends upon nutrition more than on any other single factor. – Dr. Wm. H. Sebrell, Jr.

ACV Relieves Chronic Fatigue

My father was a splendid farmer and many times I would watch him add ACV to the feed and water of ailing animals (cattle, horses, sheep, dogs, cats, etc.) and it acted like magic. ACV seemed to possess some miracle ingredient that helped restore health to the animals.*

The nearest doctor was 32 miles from our home. If a doctor was needed, he had to come by horse and buggy over miles of rough, dirt roads. So, at our home we developed simple self-health remedies and apple cider vinegar played an important health role.

I remember when my father would put in long hours at the farm during the harvest period. He was up long before daybreak and didn't retire until late at night. I would watch him come into the kitchen, put 2 heaping tsps. of honey in a glass, add 2 tsps. of raw apple cider vinegar, fill the glass with water and then sip it slowly.

I would ask, "Father, why do you drink apple cider vinegar, honey and water?" Father would reply, "Son, farm work is long, hard work. It can produce extreme body fatigue. Whatever is in this apple cider vinegar and honey drink relieves me of that chronic fatigue."

Father was definitely correct. There was an ingredient in that drink that renewed his vitality and relieved him of the chronic fatigue and stiffness. That ingredient was potassium, along with the powerful enzymes, minerals and trace elements that are in organic, raw apple cider vinegar.

Most people today, when they work hard, turn to all kinds of dangerous stimulants to relieve their chronic fatigue: alcohol, tea, coffee, cola drinks and pep pills and other dangerous, addictive drugs.

My father's good advice fell on youthful ears. It was some years later that I realized that my father was a smart man in using raw honey and raw apple cider vinegar, rich in potassium, to combat chronic fatigue.

*ACV helps animals stay healthy. Mixture: *1 cup ACV with 3 cups distilled water. Once daily in feed or water: for small animals, add 1 tsp. ACV mixture; for large animals, add 2 to 3 tsps. Or administer orally with eye dropper, baster or squeeze bottle. To relieve skin rashes or itching apply topically. Add to bath or rinse water to keep skin healthy and ward off fleas.*

Unhealthy Diet Brings Sickness

At 12, I was sent from my rugged farm life to an expensive military academy as a gift for saving a wealthy man from drowning. That institution's food gradually broke my health! The unhealthy diet of sugared, refined, overcooked and dead foods served there ruined my health. It made me the victim of a consuming disease, tuberculosis.

At no time did I see our wonderful ACV or raw honey at the table of the military academy. It was not until I met the great healer Dr. Rollier at his health sanitarium in Switzerland, where I regained my health, that I again came in contact with the miracles of ACV and *honey, both rich in essential potassium!

I owe much of my recovery to apple cider vinegar and honey, as they are persistent fighters against germs and toxins! Each morning, I was given the same drink my father took for energy and health. Dr. Rollier urged us to put apple cider vinegar on all of our raw vegetable salads and steamed greens. He also urged us to eat an abundance of raw vegetables and fresh fruits each day as they are Mother Nature's purifiers. He was a wise doctor and knew how valuable potassium and raw fruits and vegetables are for maintaining 100% health.

I was 100% cured from TB in less than 2 years after cleansing and rebuilding myself with a balanced natural diet, correct deep breathing and Alpine sunshine. Healthy living was my cure! I have been an ardent user of organic, raw ACV and raw honey ever since. In our Bragg health teachings and writings we have always advocated the use of this miraculous source of potassium.

It was in Switzerland that I started to fulfill my earlier pledge to God, that if I recovered my health, I would become a health crusader and devote my life to sharing the message of health and wellness with the world! When I finished my schooling, I went on to full-time crusading for a healthier world!

---

* *Raw honey,* used for centuries, has many miraculous nutrients and health properties. Egyptian ancient medical documents (Smith Papyrus, 2400 B.C.) recognized honey as an essential natural cure-all, listing 500 honey remedies. Hippocrates, the father of medicine, prescribed honey to his patients, and Pliny the Elder said honey was essential for good health and a long life.

Body Signs of Potassium Deficiency

Bone and muscle aches and pains, especially lower back.

Shooting pains when straightening up after leaning over.

Dizziness upon straightening up after leaning over.

Morning dull headaches upon arising and when stressed.

The body feels heavy, tired and it's an effort to move.

Dull, faded-looking hair that lacks sheen and luster.

The scalp is itchy. Dandruff, premature hair thinning or balding may occur.

The hair is unmanageable, mats, often looks straw-like, is sometimes extremely dry and other times oily.

The eyes itch, feel sore and uncomfortable, and appear bloodshot and watery. Also, eyelids may be granulated with white matter collecting in the corners.

15

The eyes tire easily and will not focus as they should.

Loss of mental alertness and onset of confusion, making decisions difficult. The memory fails, making you forget names and places you should remember.

You tire physically and mentally with the slightest effort.

You become easily irritable and impatient with your family, friends and loved ones, and even with your business and social acquaintances.

You feel nervous, depressed and in a mental fog. You have difficulty getting things done, due to mental and muscle fatigue. The slightest effort can leave you upset and trembling.

At times, your hands and feet get chilled, even in warm weather, which is also a sign of potassium deficiency.

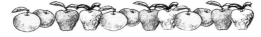

Potassium is the key mineral in the constellation of minerals;
it's so important to every living thing that without it there would
be no life. Raw apple cider vinegar is a rich source of potassium.

Life is Thrilling When You Can Help Others!

I founded the health movement and originated, named and started the first Health Food Store. Then, through The Bragg Health Crusades, I inspired hundreds of Bragg students to open the first Health Food Stores in their areas across America and then worldwide. It's thrilling and rewarding to live a life of service helping and inspiring others to live a healthy lifestyle! God has blessed me!

Apple Cider Vinegar for Overweight

More than a third of Americans are trying to lose weight. Thirty billion dollars are spent yearly on diet programs and products. Rather than a yo-yo diet, these people need The Bragg Healthy Lifestyle for life! Please understand that ACV will not reduce a person who does not control their intake of food. But the ACV drink and a healthy diet of 1,200 calories daily, plus regular exercise will assist in reducing excess weight. Also the Diet Research Center in England reported, *"better reducing and firming with ACV daily massages* (mix 3 parts ACV to 1 part almond or olive oil); helps the body reduce excess fat."* The ACV drink should be taken 3 times daily. It consists of 1 to 2 tsp. equally of organic raw ACV and raw honey (optional) mixed in a glass of distilled water.

Along with this healthy ACV drink, there must be a healthy reducing diet. (Read the Bragg *Miracle of Fasting* book for more reducing info). This means that all refined, processed, sugared products and beverages and all dairy products are eliminated from your diet. The diet should consist of a wide variety of fresh fruits; raw salads; raw nuts and seeds; raw, steamed, baked or stir-fried vegetables; brown rice; tofu; beans; and whole grain pastas. Read our Bragg Recipe book for hundreds of delicious, healthy recipes, available most health & book stores, call & request them. If unavailable call (800)446-1990.

Massages bring many beneficial healthy changes to the body: They unclog the body forces and promote circulation flow that brings healing, new feelings and smoother muscles leading to more vital health! Our inner and outer problems often hit us in the "gut" and muscles. Massages are healing, soothing and relaxing. See pages 91 to 94 for various health therapies and massages.

Combatting Underweight

Apple cider vinegar is proving to be one of the greatest aids to health known to science. It's a 100% natural substance produced by powerful natural enzymes from healthy organic apples, free of any chemicals.

The underweight person is usually deficient in these powerful enzymes and therefore cannot use or burn up the food that is put into their body. No matter how much fatty food, protein or any other kind of food is ingested, often it is not used properly by the body if important enzymes are missing. Enzyme deficiencies always cause problems! If underweight, drink the following ACV cocktail each morning upon arising: 1 tsp. ACV and 1 tsp. honey in a glass of distilled water. Add to this 2 drops of liquid iodine made from seaweed, available in Health Food Stores. This adds natural iodine, which is so important to body health and helps normalize body weight up or down as needed. Then, with each meal take a multi-digestive enzyme and always be faithful to The Bragg Healthy Lifestyle. Remember, healthy foods are needed body fuel.

Purify Your Cells by Ridding
The Body of Dangerous Toxic Wastes

Toxic poisons are the cause of most troubles in the human body. Most people do not have sufficient vital force to supply the eliminative organs with the strength to remove normal waste from the body. The toxins remain and lodge in the joints and organs of the body. We have a name for each symptom that gives us pain and trouble. Certain toxic wastes that are harmful to the whole body are rendered harmless by a miraculous substance in organic, raw ACV with the powerful *mother*. Scientists call this protective action *acetolysis*.

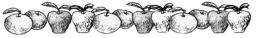

A recent study showed people with large waistlines had shorter lifespans.

Caution: The Army Diet - what you overeat goes to the front.

All the flowers of all the tomorrows are in the seeds of today.

Apple Cider Vinegar for Body Purification

It's time for life changes when you feel badly and don't seem to have the Human Go Power and Vital Force to do the things in life that are necessary! It's time to flush out the energy depleting, problem causing toxic wastes that are clogging your machinery and organs of elimination! Waste products broken down by this ACV process are flushed out. Remember, your important organs of elimination are the bowel, the lungs, the skin and the kidneys. They are your faithful servants! They work hard 24 hours a day flushing out toxic wastes. Many times these eliminative organs need help and that is when the ACV drink comes to their aid!

Follow the ACV daily program. In addition, add 1 tsp. ACV to 6 ounces of salt-free tomato or fresh vegetable juice (carrot and greens) and drink between meals, daily. Be sure to do a cleansing fast 1 day weekly and always faithfully follow The Bragg Healthy Lifestyle, which is explained throughout the book in full, simple details.

Apple Cider Vinegar Relieves Headaches

People blame their headaches on many different organs of the body. Most headaches are blamed on the eyes, the nerves, the liver, the sinuses, the stomach, the bowel, kidneys or allergies. Headaches can be put into two different classifications:

One type of chronic headache can be associated with long-standing disease. The headache is the alarm messenger telling the person that deep down in their body, destruction is going on. Pain and headaches are Mother Nature's great red flashing warning signal to take fast action! There may be trouble anywhere throughout the body. It could be in the liver, gallbladder, kidneys, bowel or any of the body's organs. It may be related to or caused by sensitive sinus, allergy or mucus problems.

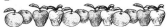

Spread love everywhere you go: first of all in your own house. Give love to your children, to your wife or husband, to a next door neighbor . . . Let no one ever come to you without leaving better and happier. Be the living expression of God's kindness; kindness in your face, kindness in your eyes, kindness in your smile, kindness in your warm greeting. – Mother Teresa

The **second type** of headache is emotional! This is often caused by nervousness, anxiety, stress, strain, tension or any personal or emotional upsets. This is a world where we must be associated with other human beings. Our daily life with others can throw us into many upsetting emotional problems because they can arouse our emotions of fear, jealousy, envy, hate, greed, self-pity or self-indulgence. When emotions reach a boiling point, we usually end up with a dull, throbbing headache. The worst type of headache is the migraine, which causes the sufferer to feel as if their head is splitting apart. Please read the Bragg book on *Nerve Force* which shows you how to be the captain of your life, health and your Nerve's precious Vital Force.

We have found in our many years of research on all kinds of headaches that when the body triggers a headache, the urine is alkaline rather than the normal acid. The kidneys are disturbed by the emotions and it means the body is off-balance. The fast working malic acid of ACV can help relieve headaches by aiding the kidneys to return the urine to normal acidity.

Vaporized ACV can also help relieve headaches. In a vaporizer or small pan, put 2 Tbsps. ACV and 2 cups distilled water. Bring mixture to a boil. When vapor begins to rise, turn heat off, put a towel over your head and lean forward over the steam, taking 5 deep breaths of the ACV mixture. Many chronic headache sufferers have told us they get blessed relief in 35 to 40 minutes with this method. In fact, they have said that after following The Bragg Healthy Lifestyle along with the ACV vapor method, they had no need for commercial headache remedies and pain killers!

Ten Little, Two-Letter Words Of Action:
IF IT IS TO BE – IT IS UP TO ME!

Simplify – Simplify – Simplify Your Life!
Streamline and unclutter your home and closets, your business and your office, your professional life and your personal life of all unnecessary baggage and things. This will help unburden your life. Now live life simpler and stay close to Mother Nature and God!
– Patricia Bragg

Apple Cider Vinegar for Feet – Combatting Corns, Callouses and Warts

For Corns and Callouses: First soak affected areas in warm water with ⅓ cup ACV for 20 to 30 minutes. After soaking, rub areas briskly with a coarse towel, then gently use a pumice stone. Now apply a full-strength ACV-soaked gauze bandage overnight, and in the morning prepare a fresh ACV soaked bandage for daytime use. These treatments help soften and dissolve corns and callouses. Check your shoes for comfort and fit. Wrong shoes are the main cause of corns, callouses, bunions and blisters. For casual wear, Birkenstock shoes are great!

Give yourself weekly pedicures, massages and also exercise your feet daily. Doing this while watching TV is ideal. Treat yourself to foot reflexology therapy (see page 92). Walking barefoot on sand, grass and at home is beneficial. Be good to your feet – they carry you through life! We kept Dr. Scholl, the famous foot doctor, going strong and alert for almost 100 years! Dr. Scholl said . . .

"**The Bragg *Health Books and Foot Book* are the best!**"

For Common Warts: Use the ACV treatment, but caution*: do not rub warts, as this could spread them!* After soaking, use ACV-soaked gauze bandage and keep it on overnight. In the morning, for daytime treatment, apply a castor oil-soaked gauze bandage. At night you can alternate ACV with crushed fresh garlic and vitamin E (prick open capsule). Combination treatments work wonders! If warts become a problem, some doctors freeze them with liquid nitrogen. This method is fast, easy and leaves no scars.

Apple Cider Vinegar Zaps Sore Throat & Laryngitis

Organic, raw ACV is a dangerous enemy to all kinds of germs that attack the throat and mouth! To fight the germs and keep the throat healthy, an ACV gargle mixture works miracles (1 tsp. to ½ glass of water). Gargle 3 mouthfuls of mixture each hour, then spit it out. Don't swallow the gargled mixture, because ACV acts like a sponge, drawing out throat and mouth germs and toxins.

As the throat feels better, gargle every 3 hours. We have famous singers from the Metropolitan Opera to Rock and Roll bands, etc. from ageless, dynamic 6'7" Jerome Hines to the eternally youthful Beach Boys, using ACV to keep their throats healthy and germ-free. It's important for singers, teachers, ministers, public speakers and you.

Along with the gargling, we use an ACV wet compress as follows: first, place a thin ACV-soaked cloth over throat area, cover with Saran Wrap, then use a flat hot water bottle or moist, hot wrung-out towel to heat the area, allowing ACV to absorb through the skin. This ACV hot compress is also great for cleansing and healing the chest area when treating all lung congestions – colds, flu, bronchitis, emphysema and asthma. It feels good, too.

Even in good health, use ACV gargle twice weekly to remove any body toxins being eliminated through the throat tissues. The gargle is also helpful during fasting, when the throat may produce a stringy mucus as part of the detoxifying process! Read our *Miracle of Fasting* book: it contains the powerful health message of fasting to detox, cleanse and renew the body.

Apple Cider Vinegar for Healthy Skin

Reap vitality with the apple cider vinegar massage: To a small basin of warm water, add ½ cup of ACV. Dip both hands in the mixture and massage this all over the nude body (in shower or bathtub): face, neck, chest, arms, shoulders, back, abdomen, legs and feet. Rub the mixture into the skin thoroughly. Be vigorous in your massage, but gentle on the face. Healthy skin has an acid reaction, for it is throwing off toxic poisons through its billions of pores. (We often call skin the third kidney.)

After thoroughly wetting the skin with the mixture several times, rub and massage until the skin is dry. Do this at least twice a week and do not wash it off; leave it on the body. As you massage the mixture into the skin, you will feel a new vitality coming into your body.

Don't Recycle Body Mucus!
Your body's machinery works hard to collect the mucus and then push it out your nose and mouth. So, when it's ready to get out – spit – cough – blow it out! Never recycle mucus by swallowing it!

The reason this treatment is far better than using soap is because soap has an alkaline reaction on the skin and you don't want that! By keeping the skin in an acid reaction, it will help you have healthier skin. I've never used soap on my face or body, just ACV and it's worked wonders. If you want to use soap – Castile soap is best.

We find after hard exercise or long mental work that we get a new feeling of strength and energy after one of these ACV massages. Also try gently dry brushing your skin with a loofah pad or vegetable brush the next time you feel mentally or physically tired and worn out. We assure you that you'll want to do it often. The health benefits of improved circulation speak for themselves!

Apple Cider Vinegar for Skin Problems

To open the pores and loosen dirt and grease from your face, turn off heat under a pan of steaming ACV water (3 Tbsp. ACV to a quart of water). Steam your face over the pan and use a towel draped over the head to trap the steam. Then pat ACV on face with a cotton ball to remove the loosened dirt. Repeat steaming and cleansing twice. Then you can gently squeeze out any blackheads. Then pat or spray on chilled ACV, diluted with an equal amount of distilled water (store ACV mixture in refrigerator) to close pores and tone the skin. Do steam cleansing twice weekly, as needed. Another excellent cleanser and toner is aloe gel or fresh aloe vera cactus pulp. Cut off 1 inch of aloe vera rib, slit open and rub yellowish pulp directly on the skin. We grow our own aloe plants – you can grow them in pots also. Aloe is a great healer for burns, pimples, sores, bites, etc!

Apple Cider Vinegar for Sunburns

Gently pat undiluted ACV on skin to give relief from sunburn. Leave it on to help prevent blistering and peeling. For all-over sunburns, pour 1 cup of ACV in cool bath water, then enjoy the healing soak. After soaking, gently dry your body, then pat on ACV to needed areas. Wait 5 minutes, then pat on aloe vera gel. For serious burns, please consult your health practitioner.

Younger Looking Skin in Minutes
With Apple Cider Vinegar Facial

The skin consists of microscopically small, flat scales that constantly flake off, thereby revealing the new skin beneath the outer, older layer of scales. In millions of people, the old, tired, dead, dry outer scales do not peel off promptly, slowing new growth and leaving their skin dry, sallow, dull and lifeless. This is known as "the old-age look."

Use this ACV facial for rejuvenating results! First, wash the skin in warm water (no soap). Next, apply a wrung-out, hot water-soaked cloth to the face for 3 minutes, then remove. Soak thin cloth in warm ACV water (2 Tbsp. ACV per cup of water) and again apply to face. Cover the ACV-soaked cloth with a towel wrung out in hot water. Relax and lie down for 10 minutes or longer with your feet elevated on couch, against a wall, or use a slant board or an ironing board. This brings more blood circulation to the face for cell rejuvenation.

Remove both cloths and gently rub skin upwards with a coarse towel or our favorite – a small loofah face pad. This rub removes the hundreds of old, dry skin scales that have been detached and loosened by the ACV facial. You can repeat this weekly or as needed. Your skin will look more youthful and will shine like a polished apple with joyous new life. We should all have pride in looking our best and presenting a good personal appearance. You will be truly amazed and proud of yourself with the results from these age-reversing, simple health treatments!

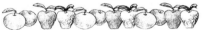

We must always change, renew, rejuvenate ourselves; otherwise, we harden. – Johann W. Goethe

God gave his creatures light and air and water open to the skies; Man locks him in a stifling lair and wonders why his brother dies. – Oliver Wendell Holmes

Prayer is the mortar that holds our house together. – Sister Teresa, James 5:16

Love is the cement that binds families together, but it is friendship that makes them happy – William Hazlitt

Skin Problems and Treatments

ACV can be used to effectively relieve the pain and discomfort of **cold sores and genital sores** caused by the herpes virus. Apply ACV directly to the affected areas and the itching and burning discomfort will rapidly dissipate. ACV also helps the sores to heal more quickly.

Shingles and chicken pox, caused by herpes zoster virus, can be relieved with straight ACV applications. Gently apply to the itching and burning areas. A cup of ACV in a warm bath will also help soothe itching.

ACV relieves the itching and discomfort caused by **poison ivy and poison oak** and other poisonous plants. Mix equal parts of ACV and distilled water and spray on the affected areas to stop the pain, itching and ease the redness and swelling. Keep spray mixture in refrigerator; a cold spray is more soothing. (Read bottom of page 25.)

Healing is faster for **minor cuts and abrasions**, and there is less chance of infection if you swab areas with ACV once a day. ACV also helps stop bleeding by helping the blood to clot. Soak a cotton ball in ACV and press on abrasion until bleeding stops.

Varicose veins can be unsightly and painful, but applications of ACV can help shrink the veins. Wrap an ACV-dampened cloth around needed areas both morning and night, then elevate legs, leaving on for 15 minutes (follow instructions on page 23). Then remove wrap, legs still up – start at ankles to gently press over pooled veins to get blood back into circulation. To help speed up the inner cleansing and healing, remember to drink and enjoy your Bragg ACV cocktail 3 times daily.

Relief from **dry, itchy skin and hives** will come after applying a paste of ACV and cornstarch to affected areas. The ACV paste mixture draws out the itching as it dries.

Oily skin can be helped by the ACV drink and the facial treatment twice a week, explained on page 23.

To help prevent **windburn, sunburn and chapping** coat the exposed skin with a 50/50 ACV and olive or avocado oil mixture. When in the elements, carry mixture along.

ACV For Insect Stings, Bites, Yeast and Fungus Problems

ACV helps stop the pain and itching from **mosquito and other insect bites, bee stings** and also neutralizes the **jellyfish's painful stinging venom**. Use straight ACV on affected areas or with a compress as often as needed. ACV also helps relieve **swimmer's ear,** a condition from swimming and showering, which also may cause temporary loss of hearing and ear infections. Dilute ACV with equal parts distilled water and drop into the ear after swimming or if you feel a blockage in your ears after showering. Drug stores stock ear dropper syringes. If infection persists, see a health professional.

Yeast and fungus infections of the body and mucus membranes (such as **thrush** in the mouth and throat, on genital areas on males and females – especially children – such as **diaper rash** and **jock itch, athlete's foot** and **eczema**) can all be treated with a 50/50 solution of ACV and distilled water. For athlete's foot, soak feet in 50/50 mixture of ACV and lukewarm water twice daily; for mouth thrush, gargle every 3 hours with 2 tsp. ACV in glass of warm water. Also slowly drink a warm Bragg ACV cocktail morning and night. For genital areas, especially in the case of itch or diaper rash* on infants, swab affected area carefully with a solution of 2 Tbsps. ACV to 1 quart warm distilled water 3 times daily. The treatments for all yeast infections should continue for at least 10 days or until symptoms dissipate.

The true physician will be a teacher; his work will be to keep them well, instead of trying to heal them after sickness. – Ralph W. Trine

---

Fixing Life's Flats: *When your life seems a bit flat, look around for a source of leakage! Life habits, actions, words, deeds, thoughts - are they healthy and happy? Just a little leak will in time cause a tire to go flat, also your life! Check your life for leaks and stop them now! – Patricia Bragg*

You will increase your health, joy, energy and peace of mind with more exercise and deep breathing every day.

---

*If it persists, try aloe vera or calendula, comfrey or zinc oxide ointments for healing of rashes on humans – babies, children, adults – and animals.

Apple Cider Vinegar for Dandruff, Itching Scalp, Dry and Thinning Hair and Baldness

The high acidity (organic malic acid) plus the powerful enzymes (the "mother's" life chemicals) in ACV kill the bottle bacillus, a germ responsible for many scalp and hair conditions. The problems caused by this are dandruff, itching scalp, thinning hair and often baldness.*

Every hair has its own oil can. Bottle bacilli can clog these tiny openings. Scales and small dry crusts are formed, resulting in itching and dandruff. The oil-starved hairs either fall out or break off, causing thinning of the hair and often baldness. ACV not only kills bottle bacillus, but stimulates the oil cans to a healthier, more balanced activity.

Pour 3 Tbsps. ACV in cup – part the hair in sections and sponge ACV directly onto scalp and wrap head with a towel. For dry hair weekly apply castor oil or olive oil to hair, and ACV to scalp, then wrap. Leave on for 30 minutes or up to 3 hours before shampooing. The ACV helps to restore the proper acid/alkaline balance to the scalp. For acute cases, do daily or before every shampoo. To promote hair growth in bald and thinning areas – rub on ACV, then royal jelly. Some people are getting great results.

For a healthy after-shampoo rinse, and for more shine and body add $\frac{1}{3}$ cup ACV to a quart of rinse water. I pre-mix it in a plastic bottle and keep it in the shower.

For Muscle Soreness and Aching Joints

To soothe tired, aching muscles and joints, there is nothing like an ACV bath combined with a self-massage. While soaking in a warm bath with 1 cup ACV added, massage the entire body, starting with the feet. Gently but firmly squeeze and relax each part of the foot, working slowly up the right leg to the hip, then the left leg. Continue up the torso, arms and neck, always rubbing toward the heart. For the face, lightly stroke skin in upward direction; avoid pulling facial skin down. Finish with a firm fingertip dry massage in circular motions over the scalp, then finger rub your ears.

---

* The Bragg Hair book gives complete hair care. Jheri Redding (founder of Nexxus and Redken) and Vidal Sassoon are long-time Bragg followers.

How to Strengthen the Heart

Enjoy your basic 3 ACV cocktails daily! Plus have another ½ tsp. ACV in ½ glass of distilled water, twice daily between meals, ideal before brisk walk or exercise.

The heart, a large muscle and your master pump uses large amounts of potassium to keep going strong for your entire life! It's the hardest working muscle in the body (see page 6). It must have a constant, continuous supply of power and energy to continue beating. ACV contains a natural chemical that combines with heart fuel to make the heart muscle stronger and helps normalize blood pressure and cholesterol. To help arrhythmia also take magnesium orotate supplements.

Low Fat Meals Cut Heart Disease Risk

A great British research report by Dr. George Miller of Britain's Medical Research Council stated: *"High fat meals make the blood more prone to clot within 6 to 7 hours after eating. Low fat meals can almost immediately reverse this condition. Most heart attacks occur in the early morning. One reason may be the overnight clotting effects of a high fat dinner. Researchers feel that by cutting fats from your diet, you may be able to add years to your life and cut the risk of heart disease!"* The University of Chicago's research supports Dr. Miller's statement that the healthy heart, low fat vegetarian meals with ample fresh fruits and vegetables are the best and safest. (See Healthy Heart Habits page 87.)

How to Improve the Digestion

Millions have indigestion, which is aggravated by poor digestion and weak saliva juices. This causes stomach distress: gas, heartburn, burping and stomach bloating. Before mealtime, sip ⅓ tsp. ACV. Hold in mouth for a minute before swallowing. This promotes enzymes and saliva, which helps start the digestion in the mouth. This causes stomach digestive fluids to flow faster, resulting in improved digestion and better health.

Organic raw apple cider vinegar with the mother is vital to the body's digestive balance by stimulating the flow of precious enzymes and saliva in the mouth. I recommend for improved digestion, sipping ⅓ tsp. before each meal to activate the flow of digestive juices.
– Gabriel Cousens, M.D., Author, *Conscious Eating*

Chewing Gum Causes Stomach Problems

Please never chew gum because it fools the body into thinking food is coming and causes precious digestive juices to start flowing. These powerful juices can cause trouble with your empty stomach's lining, resulting in ulcers, stomach problems, heart burn, bloating, gas, etc.

Fight Kidney and Bladder Problems

Avoid all animal, dairy, salt, alcohol and sugar products. All ages should follow The Bragg Healthy Lifestyle for health. Use ACV on salads and have your ACV drink 3 times daily. ACV can help bladder problems and dissolve some types of stones. Drink 8 glasses of distilled water, plus some organic, unsweetened cranberry juice. Add ⅓ tsp. ACV to each glass, which helps acidify urine, inhibits bacterial growth and promotes healing. You may sweeten the cranberry drink with organic grape juice or raw honey. You can also do a 2 or 3 day watermelon only flush. Thoroughly chew and swallow the seeds, too.

This is a great kidney – bladder cleanser and healer.

For bedwetting: Mix ½ to 1 tsp. buckwheat honey with ½ tsp. ACV before bedtime. It's best to stop liquids 3 hours before bedtime, except for small sips.

For all kidney and bladder problems: Children and adults should drink 8 glasses daily of distilled water. It's important for the urinary tract and kidneys. Use this healing and cleansing drink: 2 Tbsp *fresh or dried corn silk to 1 quart distilled water or try marshmallow herbal tea, 2 to 3 times daily. Add ½ tsp. ACV to each cup and sweeten with 1 tsp. buckwheat honey. (* Save and dry corn silks from fresh corn and store in an airtight bottle.)

To soothe and heal bladder infections: Add 1 cup ACV to warm low sitz bath. Use 1 to 2 times daily. Also, ACV douches help (page 30). Use a dipstick tester from the drugstore to check for any urinary infection.*

To eliminate "dribbles": To keep the bladder and sphincter muscles tightened and toned – urinate – stop – urinate – stop, 6 times, twice daily when voiding. This simple exercise works. After age 40, do this every day.

Important: We don't endorse antibiotics, but if you are ever on them, please take acidophilus liquid or capsules to replace the friendly bacteria in your body.

Apple Cider Vinegar Combats Gallstones

Before starting the 2 day gallbladder flush, prepare for 1 week by drinking slowly – upon arising, at mid-morning, mid-afternoon and after dinner – ½ tsp ACV with a 6 ounce glass of apple juice; or if hypoglycemic or diabetic, dilute with half distilled water. Organic, unfiltered apple juice is rich in malic acid, potassium, pectins and enzymes. These act as solvents to soften and help remove debris (small stones, etc.) and cleanse the body. Doctors have non-surgical methods for removing the difficult, larger stones using sound waves. But it's best to purge small and medium-sized ones twice yearly. These are the ones that can grow to cause problems!

No food is eaten (only liquids) during the following 2 day gallbladder flush. Combine in 8 oz glass: ⅓ virgin olive oil (no substitutes), ⅔ apple juice (organic) and 1 tsp. ACV. Drink this mixture 3 times the first day. *At night, sleep on your right side when on flush, pulling right knee toward chest to open pathway.* On the second day, take mixture twice. On both days drink all the apple juice desired, but no other liquid, not even water. This is not recommended for diabetics unless supervised by a health expert.

About midmorning on the third day, eat a raw variety salad (nature's broom) of cabbage, carrots, celery, beets, tomatoes, sprouts and lettuce, with lots of ACV and olive oil. If desired, have a bowl of lightly steamed greens, such as kale, collards, chard or other leafy greens. Season with ACV, olive oil, brewer's yeast flakes and a spray of Bragg Aminos – this gives delicious flavor to all greens.

We take this miracle cleanser flush at least once or twice a year. Check your bowel movements for tiny, greenish-brown stones. It will amaze you what your gallbladder, stomach and colon will flush out!

Everyone should be his own physician.
We ought to assist and not force nature. – Voltaire

Nature, time and patience are the three great physicians. – Irish Proverb

---

Happiness is not being pained in body or troubled in mind.
– Thomas Jefferson, Third U.S. President

Note: Some nausea may occur. This shows toxins, mucus and bile are being dumped in the stomach. Your body wants it out! If nauseated, your body is saying: "Drink 1 to 2 glasses of distilled water and regurgitate until stomach is empty." (You might have to depress your tongue while leaning over the bowl.) Once it's out, you will feel better right away! Remember, it's a wise decision when you are nauseated to get out whatever is causing your upset stomach!

Apple Cider Vinegar Helps Shrink Prostate

With a fork, "whip" 2 Tbsp. ACV with 2 Tbsp. olive oil, a dash of Bragg Liquid Aminos and cinnamon. Use this ACV mixture daily over salads, sliced tomatoes, avocados and steamed veggies. Remember, zinc and saw palmetto supplements are also healing for the prostate. Raw pumpkin seeds are rich in zinc – enjoy with meals.

Apple Cider Vinegar for Female Troubles

For a healthier vagina, use ACV douches and baths when needed, as the acidity is the same as the vagina.

Douche mixture: 3 Tbsps. ACV to 2 quarts warm distilled water is a cleansing, healing douche. If discharge is present, use 1 to 2 times daily, but less frequently as discharge lessens. **For bath:** Add 2 cups ACV to water.

To shrink, tighten and tone a flabby womb, eat raw garden salads made with extra parsley and celery. Sprinkle salads with ACV, virgin olive oil and a spray of Bragg Liquid Aminos over the top. Also exercise daily.

Fight Arthritis with Apple Cider Vinegar

Hard, stony deposits fill up, cement, enlarge and cripple the joints! Crippling, painful arthritis and joint problems are the sad result! Flush out those stony deposits with your daily ACV drinks. Upon arising, an hour before lunch and dinner have your delicious ACV cocktail as follows: Stir 6 ounces distilled water with 1 to 2 tsp. equally of ACV and raw honey (diabetics, don't use honey). Also add ACV to your salads and steamed greens. Be faithful to The Bragg Healthy Lifestyle and your 24 hour fasts. Eat 60% to 70% healthy, raw foods (organic is best) and drink

8 glasses daily of pure distilled water (chemical and inorganic mineral free). Take your multi-vitamin-mineral and glucosamine sulfate supplements, plus kelp and alfalfa tablets and 1 to 2 tsps. of cod liver oil every day. The improvements will amaze you! Remember to enjoy 1 to 2 organic apples a day for they help keep the doctor away!

Apple Cider Vinegar Combats Mucus

Millions have postnasal drip and are plagued with toxic mucus in their sinus cavities, nose and throat, which is most uncomfortable! If mucus sufferers remove all dairy products, eggs and sugars from their diet, follow The Bragg Healthy Lifestyle, take a weekly 24-hour fast and use ample ACV, soon these mucus conditions will vanish on this healthy toxicless and mucusless diet!

Upon arising, have a glass of warm, distilled water with 1 to 2 tsp. ACV and 1 to 2 tsp. raw honey. Also enjoy this drink midmorning and mid-afternoon. On your daily salads use 1 to 2 tsp. ACV combined with olive oil and a dash or spray of Bragg Liquid Aminos. Try our delicious, all-purpose Bragg Aminos in the handy, small spray bottle. This is a great method for seasoning salads, potatoes, vegetables, etc., and even popcorn! The spray bottle is perfect to take along when dining out!

For throat gargle and nasal wash: Add 1-2 tsp. ACV to ½ glass warm water for throat gargle (page 20) or nasal sniff wash to help clean out the mucus. Sniff up nostril, roll head back, then side to side, lean over, blow out mucus. Then repeat with other side. Do twice daily until mucus conditions subside. Along with the ACV drink, enjoy fresh carrot and green juices between meals. It's important to sip and savor fresh juices slowly, as they are really foods, not just beverages. Small amounts of juice (or food) in the mouth at one time will be better digested and more easily used by the body chemistry.

ACV mouthwash: (1 tsp ACV to glass water) Kills mouth bacteria, fights plaque and tartar, helps prevent gum disease, promotes healing and freshens the breath.

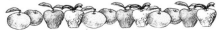

At mealtime come thou hither and eat of the bread
and dip the morsel in the vinegar. – Ruth 2:14

For Nosebleeds

Soak a cotton ball or gauze in ACV and lightly pack in nostrils. Relax, sit down and lean forward for 10 minutes (breathe through mouth) pressing nostrils together while ACV pack helps blood congeal. Repeat if needed. Vitamins C and K are helpful. Be sure to drink 8 glasses of distilled water daily – nosebleeds are often caused by dehydration.

Apple Cider Vinegar and Constipation

It's important that the bowels move regularly and freely. Outgo should equal intake. You should have a bowel movement soon after arising and within an hour after meals. Flaxseed tea with ACV acts as a bowel lubricant, as do fresh fruits, vegetables and distilled water.

Make the ACV-Flaxseed Bowel Lubricant Mixture: Boil two cups distilled water and 4 Tbsps. flaxseeds (rich in Omega-3 for your heart) for 10 minutes. Mixture becomes jellylike when cool. Add 2 Tbsps. of mixture plus 1 tsp. ACV to glass of distilled water. Drink upon arising and an hour after dinner. Store mixture in the refrigerator and use as needed for good bowel movements.

Mix Half Raw Oat Bran & Half Psyllium Husk Powder: Bottle this super cleansing mixture and add 1-2 Tbsp. to any of these: ACV drink, juice, glass distilled water, herb tea or soups, etc.; let mixture soak one minute before drinking! This helps cleanse the mucus along the small intestine and colon walls and pulls toxins from the gastrointestinal tract. Also, virgin olive oil over salads, veggies, potatoes, etc., helps detoxify the colon plus adds a delicious flavor to foods.

For Easier-Flowing Bowel Movements:

Squatting is the natural way to have a bowel movement. It opens up the anal area more directly. When on the toilet, putting your feet up 6 to 8 inches on a waste basket or footstool gives you the same squatting effect. Then from behind use your fingers to gently pull up on the edge of the anus opening –this helps it roll out easier!

To check bowel elimination time: Have some fresh or frozen whole corn with your evening meal. Purposely don't chew all the kernels. (Always chew food thoroughly otherwise.) Check your stools to see when the corn is eliminated, usually within 14 hours. When it's cleansed of toxins and malnutrition is treated, the body becomes healthier and starts working more normally. Because constipation brings on many health problems, including arthritis, it's important to keep the pipes (colon and arteries) clean and open by following The Bragg Healthy Lifestyle.

The body is self-cleansing and self-healing! It is our duty if we want vibrant, glorious health to do all we can to make the body work efficiently to maintain vital, super health. Not only is a healthy diet necessary, but so are good sleeping habits, outdoor physical activity, full, deep breathing and a serene mind. We cannot live by bread alone. We must have spiritual food. We must strive for a perfect, healthy balance: physical, mental, emotional and spiritual!

What Becomes of the Acid Crystals Precipitated in the Body That Age Us?

You have often heard the expression, "He's old and stiff and his flesh is tough." When you think of "old" people you usually think of them as having stiffness in their body, with tough, brittle flesh (see Dr. Carrel's study on page 10).

Why do people get stiff in the joints and their flesh tough when they have added birthdays to their life? Most people would answer this complex question with the remark, "Because they are old." But this is not the real answer why people get stiff joints and tough flesh. The answer to premature ageing is unhealthy living and potassium deficiency. People rarely study their bodies or learn what to eat for healthy tissues and youthful joints. They are satisfied to eat what agrees with them. Or they eat foods they were reared on as children and carry these early eating habits (often unhealthy) right into their adult life and then into their children's lives!

Pray for wisdom in your daily living, for more faith and for more patience with yourself and others before you pray for just things.

Rearing Healthy Children is Important

The Bragg family children, grandchildren and great-grandchildren have all been reared on The Bragg Healthy Lifestyle. We were taught to keep in perfect health so that the body tissues would remain soft and tender and have elasticity and health. This correct way of eating enables us to come to the later years of life with youthful looking skin, keen hearing, sharp, sparkling eyes and perfect mental, emotional and physical health, for a long, useful, happy and healthy life.

Miracles with Apple Cider Vinegar

The members of the Bragg family follow The Bragg Healthy Lifestyle. They have learned the lessons of good nutrition and the miracles of ACV for themselves and their animals. The children were impressed when Farmer Bragg would have an old hen prepared for dinner. The old hen's meat was tough and didn't taste good. This is what happens to poultry and beef when it is deficient in potassium. Human flesh suffers the same problems.

To prove to the children conclusively that apple cider vinegar and honey needed to be an important part of their daily nutrition, he would then select another old hen for the dinner table. This time he fed that old hen ACV twice a day, for ten days. When the hen was prepared for the dinner table, the children tasted the difference in the old hen's meat. They noticed how tender it was – just like a young hen and they asked for second helpings. (P.S. Most of the Bragg family members are now happy, thriving, heart-healthy vegetarians!)

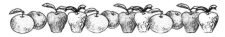

Miracles can happen everyday – through guidance and prayer!

Children are very responsive to healthy lifestyle changes, and those start with providing the right foods (fruits, vegetables, whole grains and reasonable amounts of other healthful snacks), encouraging regular exercise and activity and limiting television watching!
– Susan K. Rhodes, Ph.D., Medical University of South Carolina

A friend may well be reckoned the masterpiece of nature.
– Ralph Waldo Emerson

WE THANK THEE

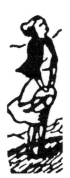

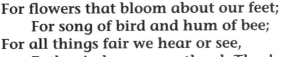

For flowers that bloom about our feet;
    For song of bird and hum of bee;
For all things fair we hear or see,
    Father in heaven we thank Thee!
For blue of stream and blue of sky;
    For pleasant shade of branches high;
For fragrant air and cooling breeze;
    For beauty of the blooming trees;
Father in heaven we thank Thee!
    For mother love and father care,
For brothers strong and sisters fair;
    For love at home and here each day;
For guidance lest we go astray,
    Father in heaven we thank Thee!
For this new morning with its light;
    For rest and shelter of the night;
For health and food, for love and friends;
    For every thing His goodness sends,
Father in heaven we thank Thee!
    – Ralph Waldo Emerson

35

Doubt destroys.
Faith builds! – Robert Collier

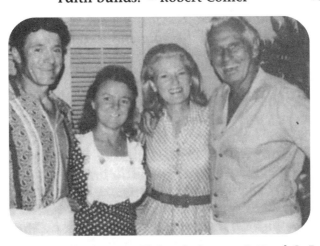

Jack LaLanne, Patricia Bragg, Elaine LaLanne & Paul C. Bragg

Jack says, "Bragg saved my life at age 15, when I attended the Bragg Health and Fitness Crusade in Oakland, California." From that day, Jack has continued to live The Bragg Healthy Lifestyle, inspiring millions to health and fitness!

All Through Your Life
You Must Fight Acid Crystals

When acid crystals harden in the joints and tissues of any animal, the joints become stiff and the tissues hardened. The meat becomes tough and tasteless. But, when the animals are given apple cider vinegar regularly, the precipitated acid crystals enter into a solution and pass out of the body, thus making the body tissues healthier and tender. This applies to human flesh also.

Now, when body tissues hold all the precipitated acid crystals they can, the crystals then appear in the bursae and the joints of the body, resulting in bursitis and arthritis. 1 to 2 tsp. of apple cider vinegar with 1 to 2 tsp. of raw honey in a glass of distilled water 3 times daily will help relieve stiff, aching, prematurely old joints. You be the judge. See how elastic and flexible all your joints become!

Keep Your Joints and Tissues Youthful

Most people have lost their normal contact with Mother Nature and simple, natural living. They no longer know how to eat the simple way God intended.

If you suffer from prematurely old joints and hardened tissues, take the ACV mixture three times daily. Eliminate or cut down on animal proteins. Stop all refined sugars, products and beverages! Then you will see how very youthful your body begins to feel.

THE HEALTH LAW OF LIFE

Man's body was created according to the laws of chemistry and physics, which are the Creator's own laws. They never vary. His law is written upon every nerve, muscle and every faculty that has been entrusted to us. These laws govern the cells, tissues and organs of the body as they carry on their various functions. They operate largely through the complex network of nerves that run throughout the body. They act through the central nervous system, from which nerve impulses originate, and through the autonomic nervous system, that part of the network not under the direct control of the will.
– Henry W. Vollmer, M.D.

Loving thoughts are little seeds . . . Let them blossom into deeds.

Roses and flowers are God's autograph.

ACV Helps Stiffness Vanish From Body

You will find, after several months of the ACV and honey cocktail taken 3 times daily – that the stiffness and misery will be gone from your joints and body. You will discover you can walk or run up several flights of stairs without any effort and pain! You will notice that you look younger and feel younger!

Make The Bragg Healthy Lifestyle a life-long daily habit! Over the years we have seen many stiff-jointed, prematurely old people transform themselves into new, youthful, healthy people! We can't do it for you. You must make the effort to give this ACV and honey program a chance to prove what it can do for you!

Questions About Apple Cider Vinegar

Many people have some preconceived idea that apple cider vinegar is harmful to the body. Instead it's the distilled, pasteurized, filtered, the malt and synthetic, dead vinegars that must be avoided for human consumption!

37

Let us assure you that there is nothing in this wonderful, organic, raw ACV that can in any way harm your body! People ask us about the merits and benefits of ACV. See the inside front cover for a list of some of the miracles it can perform.

Animal proteins and fats have a tendency to thicken the blood, while the natural acids and enzymes in ACV help to keep the blood healthier and thinner. Also, that's why people naturally crave and serve cranberry sauce, which contains four different natural acids, with turkey and other fowl. They serve applesauce with roast pork dishes and a slice of lemon with fish, or steak with mushrooms, all rich in natural acids.

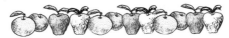

Works, not words, are the proof of love!

The use of organic apple cider vinegar is a wonderful health aid, and the #1 food I recommend in helping to maintain the body's vital acid-alkaline balance. Everyone should read this Bragg Apple Cider Vinegar *book.*
– Gabriel Cousens, M.D., Author of *Conscious Eating* and *Spiritual Nutrition*

ACV Helps Blood Pressure Become Normal

Natural food acids served along with animal proteins are designed to lessen the blood thickening influence of these heavy proteins. In order for blood to circulate freely throughout the body, it must be thin. When blood thickens, it strains the heart. The blood pressure then goes up and a host of other health problems begin.

Remember, blood has to circulate all over the body through the arteries, blood vessels and tiny capillaries. It's impossible for blood to circulate freely through these hair-like pipes when it is thickened with too many heavy protein meals, fats, hardened oils, etc.

Several years ago, we met a woman with extremely high blood pressure. We put her on a two day ACV, honey and water fast program with nothing to eat for 48 hours. She had an ACV cocktail 5 times daily, plus 4 glasses of pure distilled water – total of 9 glasses.

In 48 hours, her blood pressure had dropped to almost normal! The buzzing in her ears ceased, and her dull headache stopped. After a short period of correct eating (no salt, sugar, saturated fats, tea, coffee, etc.) combined with The Bragg Healthy Lifestyle and ACV program her blood pressure was normal and she felt reborn!

People ask us if ACV will make them slender. It helps balance the body chemistry and normalize the body weight. We have been using the ACV program in the Bragg family for over five generations and it has brought wonderful results for our health and our bodies.

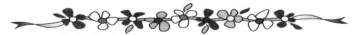

Evidence reveals that ACV has been shown to lower blood pressure and strengthen the heart muscle because it acts as a blood thinner and reduces the risk of a stroke. It contains potassium which is also vital and of great importance to the heart and blood.

The more natural food you eat, the more radiant health you will enjoy and you will be better able to promote the higher life of love and brotherhood. – Patricia Bragg

Who you are speaks so loudly, I can't hear what you're saying.
– Ralph Waldo Emerson

The Bragg Healthy Lifestyle Promotes Super Health

The Bragg Healthy Lifestyle consists of eating 60%-70% fresh, organic, live foods: raw vegetables, salads, sprouts, fresh fruits and fresh juices; raw seeds and nuts; 100% whole grain breads, pastas, cereals, nutritious beans and legumes. These are the good no cholesterol, no fat, no salt, no sugar, "live foods" – the body fuel required for lively, healthy people! This is the reason people become revitalized and reborn into a fresh, new life filled with joy, health, vitality, youthfulness and longevity! There are millions of Bragg Healthy Lifestyle followers around the world! When it works for you, please write and share your results with us, we love hearing from our readers!

Five Generations of Healthy Braggs – Thanks to All Using Apple Cider Vinegar

Since birth, all the Bragg children have used ACV. They fed it to their children and now their grandchildren are feeding it to the great-grandchildren! We all use ACV along with virgin olive oil on our salads. We put both on our steamed greens (cabbage, chard, collards, kale, spinach, mustard and beet greens, broccoli, Brussels sprouts and cauliflower) and many other foods.

Millions of our students around the world have used ACV and never once has anyone reported a negative reaction from using it. In fact, they sing its praises! So, you also will soon see the benefits from using ACV and following The Bragg Healthy Lifestyle Program.

The strongest principle of growth lies in the human choice.
– George Elliot

The body and the mind are so closely connected that not even a single word or thought can come into existence without being reflected in the personality and health of the individual. – John Prentiss

Everything is brighter in the new dawn's light –
especially after a recharging, good night's sleep!

Apple Cider Vinegar and Arthritis

People ask if ACV cures arthritis. This is not possible, for curing is an internal biological function that only the body can perform. A healthy, natural diet, deep breathing, exercise, rest, relaxation and living the Bragg Healthy Lifestyle are required to put the body in a condition to cure itself. ACV is an important part of the program (page 30). When all Mother Nature's supreme forces are used, the body will turn from sickness to wellness. Health is something you must desire, seek out, earn and always guard and treasure for your life's sake!

Apple Cider Vinegar Relieves Muscle Cramps

Many people are awakened in the middle of the night with sharp, painful muscle cramps. These often occur in the feet and lower or upper legs. Sometimes they occur in the stomach, intestines and occasionally in the heart. These are frightening experiences! Most people who experience leg cramps are forced to jump out of bed and pound or firmly massage the area to get relief. Many people with cramps in other parts of the body have to walk quickly to get relief. When precipitated acid crystals get into the circulation of the legs and other parts of the body, they can cause severe cramps.

40

We recommend taking 2 tsps. ACV and 2 tsps. of honey in a glass of distilled water three times daily to relieve these painful cramps. This allows the precipitated acid crystals to enter into a solution and pass out of the body, causing cramps to cease. Calcium and also magnesium orotate supplements taken before bedtime can also help prevent cramping, plus they promote sound sleep.

Acid Crystals Cause Premature Ageing

Everyone, even the healthiest person in the world, must continually fight the buildup of acid crystals in the body. The strongest enemy of acid crystals is the organic apple cider vinegar, raw honey and distilled water cocktail. This powerful mixture puts the acid crystals in solution so they can be flushed out of the body by the kidneys and other organs of elimination.

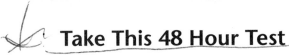

Take This 48 Hour Test

For 2 full days, take nothing into your system but liquids. Have the ACV cocktail 3 to 5 times daily, plus another 4 to 5 glasses of distilled water daily as well. Ample water is needed to flush the toxins out!

On the second and third day, after you have eaten nothing else for 48 hours, take a sample of your first early morning urine. Put these urine samples in labeled bottles with lids. Place them on a shelf and let them stand. After 2 weeks, examine sediment on the bottom of the bottles. These are some of the disease-causing toxins that were flushed out of your body!

Potassium – The Master Mineral

Always keep in mind the fact that potassium puts toxic poisons in solution so they can be flushed out of the body. **The body is self-cleansing, self-correcting, self-repairing and self-healing!** Just give it the tools to work with and you will have a painless, tireless, ageless body, regardless of your age! Forget age and calendar years, for age isn't toxic! You age prematurely when you suffer from malnutrition and potassium deficiencies. These cause low Vital Force and waste buildups – poor elimination – allowing disease to proliferate.

41

The Bragg Healthy Lifestyle will help you rebuild your Vital Force. Watch the transformation that will take place in your body when you faithfully follow your ACV regimen. You can and will create the kind of person you want to be! Plan, plot and follow through! Start now!

Although you must follow this program closely, do not try to do everything listed here immediately. Remember, it took you a long time of living by wrong habits to cause any of the problems your body might have now. So, it's going to take time for the body to cleanse, repair and rebuild itself into a more *perfect healthy home* for you! Please remember, your body is your temple while on this earth, so cherish it and protect it!

Many studies have shown that people who lower their blood cholesterol levels by diet can slow, or even reverse, atherosclerosis and cut their risk of heart attack. – University of California, Berkeley *Wellness Letter*

Please Slow Me Down Lord

Slow me down Lord and fill me with your love.

Ease the pounding of my heart by the quieting of my mind.

Quiet my hurried pace with a vision of eternal time.

Give me, amid the confusion of the day,
    the calmness of the everlasting hills.

Break the tensions of my nerves and muscles with the soothing
    music of the singing streams that live in my memory.

Help me to know the magical, restoring power of sound sleep.

Teach me the art of taking minute vacations or slowing down
    to look at a flower, to chat with a friend, to pat a dog,
    to read a few lines from a good book.

Slow me down Lord and inspire me to send my roots deep into
    the soil of life's enduring values, so that I may grow
    toward the stars of my greater destiny.

Change your mind and change your life!

Where there is no vision, the people perish. – Proverbs 29:18

*A strong body and a bright, happy or serene countenance can
only result from the fine admittance of thoughts of joy and
goodwill and serenity into the mind.* – James Allen

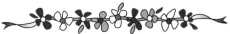

Earth laughs in flowers. – Ralph Waldo Emerson

*It never hurts to brush up on the three Rs:
Respect for yourself. Respect towards others.
Responsible living today, tomorrow and always!*

If you truly love Nature, you will find Beauty everywhere.
– Vincent Van Gogh

*A book is a garden, an orchard, a storehouse, a party, a mentor, a teacher,
a guidepost, a counsellor.* – Henry Ward Beecher

My father and I have shared The Bragg Healthy Lifestyle Blueprint with millions of people around the world at the Bragg Health and Fitness Crusades. I would now like to share it with you as part of the Apple Cider Vinegar Health System.

With Blessings of Health, Peace, Joy and Love,

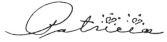

The Bragg Healthy Lifestyle

The Bragg Blueprint for Physical, Mental and Spiritual Improvement – Healthy, Vital Living to 120

– Genesis 6:3

by
Patricia Bragg, N.D., Ph.D.
Life Extension Nutritionist

Just think, in only 90 days you can build a new bloodstream! Not a thick, sluggish, toxin-saturated bloodstream, but a rich, red bloodstream, healthy in all the vitamins, minerals and vital nutrients necessary for radiant and long lasting health. First and foremost, we must build the iron content of our bloodstream. This is one of the great secrets of life: The more iron in your bloodstream, the more oxygen is going to flood into your body, purifying its cells. Oxygen is the greatest stimulant in the world. It stimulates, but does not depress. Unnatural stimulants stimulate, but there is an aftermath of depression. Tobacco, alcohol, coffee, tea, refined white sugar and drugs (prescribed and over the counter) have this bad effect on the body, but not God's own oxygen – it's the invisible staff of life!

So, in The Bragg Healthy Lifestyle we forever discard these harmful, destructive stimulants. You are going to be strong and never allow these to enter your body again! You are going to rely on the wonderful, natural stimulants to create a more healthy vital force.

Man's days shall be to 120 years. – Genesis 6:3

First, you are going to start breathing deeper and slower, as it's important for super energy. Then you are going to eat organic, live foods, such as fresh fruits and vegetables and freshly squeezed juices, that will build up your blood health and energy.

Before you eat or drink anything, I want you to ask yourself this important question, "Is this going to build a healthy bloodstream or destroy it?" Be on the alert to protect your precious river of life - your bloodstream! When it demands liquids, give it the best – pure distilled water or live-food juices, such as fresh organic fruit and vegetable juices. Get yourself a juicer. Every day fortify your bloodstream with fresh orange, grapefruit or carrot and green juices or combine different juices such as celery, tomato, beet and parsley or see page 65. Two of the best juices to add to vegetable juices are raw spinach and watercress. For a taste delight, add the juice of 1 to 2 garlic buds, an excellent purifier and heart protector.

Do not consume too much of these powerful, live-food juices. One to two pints a day is more than enough! Some people get a juicer and overdo it. Overloading your body with juices can upset your delicate blood-sugar balance. Eating the whole fruit is still the best! Just because something is good for you doesn't mean that a lot of it is. As with all things in life, moderation of your food intake is best for building Vitality Supreme!

Imagine: In just a short 11 months you will have an absolutely New You! The billions of soft cells that make up eyes, nose, skin, hands and feet, as well as all the vital organs of your body, will be renewed. You do not need to submit to the huge risk of heart, kidney or any other dangerous transplant operations!

You have within your power, through the food you eat, the liquid you drink and the air you breathe, the ability to build a fresh, vital body from the top of your head to the tip of your toes. You are what you eat and what you eat today will be walking and talking tomorrow! How wonderful our Creator has been to us, to give us the power every 90 days to build a new bloodstream and every 11 months, an entirely new body.

It's Never Too Late to Seek and Build Radiant Health!

The Creator gave us the intelligence and reasoning power to take control of our body! But the flesh is dumb! You can stuff anything in your stomach and almost get away with it until the day of reckoning!

Most young people live this way, because they believe they are totally indestructible! But what a sad lesson they learn after 40 or 50 years of wrong living! The infirmities and the aches and pains creep into their bodies, making life miserable and proving to them that their dream of indestructibility was a myth and a lie!

Live by the reasoning mind, rather than by the senses of the body. The dumb senses are constantly enticing you to do the very things that destroy your wonderful body. Look around you at the sad, broken-down human sights you see. Weak people, mentally depressed people and sickness everywhere! The average person's suffering – it's sad but true – is self-inflicted . . . a slow, self-murder!

For whatsoever a man soweth, he shall also reap. – Gal 6:7

We should know and observe the fact that everything in the universe is always governed by definite laws. If we understand and follow these universal laws we will sow the seeds of constructive, healthy living!

Make every day a healthy day and each day you will improve! You will feel new strength and energy flooding into your body. The feelings you will experience when you live The Bragg Healthy Lifestyle are indescribable! What an incredibly powerful and joyful feeling it is to be fully alive and vigorous, with unlimited energy and powerful nerve force. An amazing example is ageless Jack LaLanne who is filled with energy!

Weak people find weak excuses to continue living their unhealthy lifestyle. They will tell you they are too old to begin The Bragg Healthy Lifestyle Program. Age has no force, nor is it toxic! Time is just a measure. Long ago, the Bragg family gave up living by calendar years. We only live by biological years and we feel ageless.

Millions Suffer from Premature Ageing

There are millions in their 30s and 40s who are, sad to say, prematurely old biologically. Yet there are many people in their 70s, 80s and 90s who are biologically youthful, active, healthy and happy!

In our opinion, if you are experiencing premature ageing, you are suffering from a highly toxic condition and you are suffering from unnecessary nutritional deficiencies. These are the main causes of most human troubles. The Bragg Healthy Lifestyle will show you how to banish these vicious enemies. From this minute on, stop living by calendar years! Just forget your birthdays, as I do. All of us are reborn every second of the day as new body cells are being constantly created.

Cease this talk of getting old! From this minute on, you will have no age except your biological age and this you are going to control. Every day say to yourself . . .

"I Will Stay Youthful, Active, Happy and Healthy!"

Say it repeatedly, burn it deeply into your mind and it will sparkle all your days for your whole life!

Most people have a dreadful fear of getting old. They picture themselves half blind, hearing impaired, with teeth gone, energy and vitality spent or senile. They see themselves as a burden to their family and friends. They envision themselves in the nursing home alone, forgotten, with Alzheimer's disease.

Despite the fear of old age and the train of ailments that go with it, you can prevent this human tragedy. You can skip this terrible period by changing how you live from this day forward. Today is the day to prepare against becoming senile and decrepit. That is why I urge you to follow the wise and wonderful laws of Mother Nature. You will grow younger as you live longer! That is what this health program is all about: The preservation of your precious vital health!

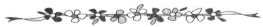

Every man is the builder of a temple called his body . . . We are all sculptors and painters and our material is our own flesh and blood and bones. Any nobleness begins at once to refine a man's features, any meanness or sensuality to imbrute them. – Henry David Thoreau

Wise Prevention Helps Keep You Healthy, Youthful and Vigorous!

Lengthening life by special treatment of chronic miseries often means merely adding years of ill health and misery to a person's life. This is often called "the living death." Who wants to extend life just to suffer? In my opinion, the true function of the healer today is to prevent sickness and disease.

No person is able to heal you! Only you can heal yourself! In order to be healthy it's essential to learn how to live healthy in order to be healthy always. They say –

An ounce of prevention is worth a pound of cure!

My father and I always stress to our readers that prevention is always the healthiest, best and is priceless!

Diet for health and youthfulness – Your diet should be composed of 60% to 70% raw fruit and raw or steamed, baked or wokked vegetables. By this habit, such conditions as stomach upsets, miseries and constipation, which occur so often in children and adults, can be avoided! Output should equal intake. You should have a bowel movement soon upon arising and after each meal.

47

The greatest enemy of health is constipation, but this can be eliminated by a diet that gives you sufficient bulk, moisture, lubrication and vigorous exercise of the entire abdominal cavity. In the remote parts of the world, where we have traveled beyond the influences of so-called modern civilization, mankind indulges in the normal habit of defecation after every meal. I want you to train yourself to have a bowel movement soon after arising and after each meal. Children can be taught this important habit from infancy. Living The Bragg Healthy Lifestyle faithfully, constipation vanishes!

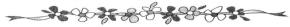

The lightest breakfast is the best. – Oswald

Why not look for the best – the best in others, the best in ourselves, the best in all life situations? He who looks for the best knows the worst is there but refuses to be discouraged by it. Though temporarily defeated, dismayed, he smiles and tries again. If you look for the best, life will become pleasant for you and everyone around you.
– Rev. Paul S. Osumi, Honolulu, Hawaii

Constipation Creates Toxins in the Body

Studies reveal the presence of toxic poisons in cases of constipation. When these toxins are absorbed into the general circulation, the liver "your detoxifying organ" is unable to cope with them. These toxins are then thrown back into the body to cause trouble and sickness. Constipation and toxemia are our real enemies!

I believe that diet plays a vital role in the maintenance of health, good elimination and the prevention of disease. Research shows that diets composed of refined white flour and sugar; preserved meats, such as hot dogs and luncheon meats; white rice; coffee, tea, cola drinks and alcohol; margarine; overcooked vegetables; high fat, sugared, salted, and processed foods create many serious health problems, especially in the intestinal tract, heart and respiratory areas. It's wise to never eat refined, processed, embalmed and dead, unhealthy foods!

Your Energy is Your Body's Spark Plug

Your energy comes from the spark of life, which is maintained by the atomic energy contained within every single cell of the human body. It embodies electrons, protons and neutrons. They are constantly discharging their ionic compounds as energy is expended in work or play, whether mental or physical, in accordance with natural laws. This energy loss must be replaced. Every cell in your body is like a battery that, when run down, must be recharged. Primarily, this is done through the intake of food. Proper breathing and exercise also helps recharge your billions of cells.

Now, there are two kinds of food: The first is in a low rate of physical vibration, like the foods we mentioned: the processed, chemicalized, dead foods, as in refined white flour and sugars, etc. It's impossible to have a youthful, dynamic body when, year after year, you feed it food and drinks with a low rate of vibration.

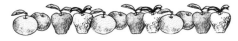

Jesus said, "Thy faith hath made thee whole, now go and sin no more." That includes your dietetic sins! He himself, through fasting and prayer, was able to heal the sick and cure all manner of diseases.

The Bragg Healthy Lifestyle Program consists only of the **second kind of foods**: those in a **high rate of vibration**. Many people have the preconceived idea that protein is the food that is in the highest rate of vibration. While protein is an important nutrient to the human body, fresh fruit has a higher rate of vibration. Fruit produces blood sugar, which helps to feed the nerves of the body. Fruit has a twofold purpose in the body. First, it's rich in blood sugar; second, it's an important, needed detoxifier and destroyer of harmful obstructions, wastes and toxins that can do the body great harm.

Allergies are Often the Body Cleansing

Often you will hear people say, "I am allergic to apples, grapefruit, peaches, strawberries, etc." These people have no idea what these foods are doing in their bodies. To give you an example, when my father was reared in the South, his typical diet was rich in animal proteins and fats from the hogs, chickens, cows and sheep they raised. At each meal, they had a wide variety of these meat proteins. I'm sad to say that accompanying these dishes were white flour biscuits and bread, mashed and fried potatoes and inevitably, a heavy, sugary dessert.

When he attended this military school (page 14) from the age of 12 on, his body became so saturated with toxic poisons, mucus and putrid food residues that, when he ate any fresh fruits, he suffered not only hives, but also colds, headaches and pains as well. These were erroneously thought to be allergic reactions. But they were the natural self-cleansing responses of his body that wanted him healthy and clean! The cleansing fruits were trying to push out the mucus and toxins through his skin, lungs, etc.!

He avoided eating these vital foods until he became a health advocate at the age of sixteen. Only after he had been cleansed and purified with healthy foods, apple cider vinegar and fasting one day a week, along with occasional longer fasts, could he eat fresh fruits and vegetables without a negative reaction.

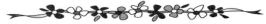

We can change if we set our will to it. – Robert Benson

Through fasting and careful nutrition, he slowly detoxified himself and could eat all the wonderful, natural foods without experiencing the allergic cleansing reactions of his youth. His early TB was the outcome of these wrong foods. For this reason, people who have been living on a diet high in animal proteins, fats, salt, starches and refined sugars can't immediately include a large amount of fresh fruits and vegetables in their diet. It's best to slowly ease into The Bragg Healthy Lifestyle to allow the body to cleanse itself gently.

Health Transition Diet - Everyone who wants to live the healthy life must thoroughly understand just what is going on in their body chemistry. Fresh, organic, raw fruits and vegetables help flush the toxins out. The body can't be rushed. It takes the average person a long time to saturate the body with toxic poisons. Now it's going to take time to flush this debris out with this transition diet!

The more organic raw fruits and raw vegetables that you condition yourself to handle, the more cleansed your body will become! So, recognize these foods, which are in the highest rate of healthy vibration. But please, also respect their cleansing and detoxifying action!

> **We often eat 100% raw meals of fruits, vegetables or salads for a few days, but usually our meals are 60% to 70% raw:**

Breakfast: Fresh, raw juice (orange, grapefruit, or carrot, celery, garlic, spinach, etc.) or raw fruit (in season, melon, apricot, berry, peach, nectarine, etc.) or the nutritious, delicious Bragg Pep Drink – recipe page 96.

Lunch: Large variety salad with fresh greens, vegetables, sprouts and a few raw nuts or seeds (sunflower, sesame, pumpkin, almonds, pecans, walnuts, etc.) See page 97.

Dinner: Variety salad, followed by two steamed, baked or wokked fresh vegetables and one of the following: beans, lentils, brown rice, whole grain pasta, tofu (soybean curd), baked or steamed potatoes.

Remember to get your daily ACV into your diet with the ACV Cocktail and sprinkle ACV over steamed greens, cauliflower, squash, broccoli, cabbage, stringbeans, etc. It is also especially delicious on garden variety salads.

People are told they must start the day with a big breakfast, to give them great energy in the morning hours. So, they gorge themselves on processed cereal with milk and sugar; ham and eggs; or bacon and eggs; stacks of hot cakes or buttered toast and jelly. All of this is washed down with coffee, milk or cocoa. You will note that there are no fresh fruits at this meal.

Only a person doing the most strenuous physical labor could possibly burn up a meal like this, and I doubt that even they would. All the vital energy of the body will be needed to digest these heavy animal proteins and fats, refined starch and white sugar breakfasts. All too often, they lie in the stomach like a ton of bricks and have to be dynamited out. Now you know why there is so much indigestion and constipation and why laxatives are one of the biggest sellers in drugstores!

So, I ask you, how in the name of common sense can a big meal like this give a person strength for their morning duties? The truth of the matter is, it can't! This is how parents and, consequently, their children are brainwashed by the big food interests who sell all their commercial, unhealthy foods.

You must change your ideas about food! Learn to eat in moderation. It's important you not overfuel your body. If you overfeed your body, you clog it up. A diet of healthy, organic, raw foods with a high rate of vibration will help keep your insides clean and healthy!

Vegetarians are Healthier and Live Longer

Most uninformed nutritionists call meat the #1 source of protein. Those proteins coming from the vegetable kingdom are referred to as the #2 proteins. This is a sad and terrible mistake. It should be the other way around! In this day and age, almost all meat is laden with herbicides, fungicides, pesticides and other chemicals that are sprayed on or poured into the feed which these animals consume. They are also pumped full of hormones, antibiotics, growth stimulators and drugs to fatten them up and keep them from dying from the unhealthy conditions they live in!

Eliminating Meat is Safer and Healthier

Play it safe, become a healthy vegetarian. Look what they feed cattle – the dead, ground up carcasses of other feed lot animals who, for a variety of reasons, didn't make it to the slaughterhouse.

Speaking of the slaughterhouse, what kind of chemical reaction do you suppose would occur in your body if somebody put a choke chain around your neck to keep you in line, shoved you onto a conveyor belt, and made you watch in horror as all of those in line in front of you were beheaded one by one? Well, your body would be pumped so full of adrenaline from all that fear you wouldn't know what hit you! Unused adrenaline is extremely toxic. If you think for a minute that most of the meat that you consume is not packed with this toxic substance, you're sadly mistaken!

Also, consider the fact that cattle, sheep, chickens, etc., are all vegetarians. When you eat them, you are just eating polluted vegetables. Why not skip all the waste and toxins and just eat healthy, organic vegetables?

And what about that myth that you have to eat meat to get your protein? If that were true, where do you suppose farm animals, especially horses, get their protein? They are vegetarians! They get their protein from the grains and grasses that they eat. You are no different. You can get the proteins you need from the large variety of whole grains, tofu, raw nuts, seeds, beans, fruits and vegetables that God put on this planet for your health. Study the Vegetable Protein % Chart.

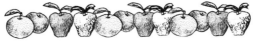

A truly good book teaches me better than to just read it. I must soon lay it down and commence living its wisdom. What I began by reading, I must finish by acting! – Henry David Thoreau

Whatsoever was the father of disease, an ill diet was the mother. – Herbert, 1859

Millions of Americans are committing slow suicide with their unhealthy, inactive lifestyle; heavy meat eating, high sugar and fat diets; plus smoking, alcohol and drugs . . . all this damages their organs and the inside of their arteries, adding more health problems to their lives! – Patricia Bragg

Vegetable Protein Percentage Chart

LEGUMES	%
Soybean sprouts	54
Mungbean sprouts	3
Soybean curd (tofu)	43
Soy flour	35
Soybeans	35
Soy sauce	33
Broad beans	32
Lentils	29
Split peas	28
Kidney beans	26
Navy beans	26
Lima beans	26
Garbanzo beans	23

VEGETABLES	%
Spinach	49
New Zealand Spinach	47
Watercress	46
Kale	45
Broccoli	45
Brussels Sprouts	44
Turnip Greens	43
Collards	43
Cauliflower	40
Mustard Greens	39
Mushrooms	38
Chinese Cabbage	34
Parsley	34
Lettuce	34
Green Peas	30
Zucchini	28
Green beans	26
Cucumbers	24
Dandelion Greens	24
Green Pepper	22
Artichokes	22
Cabbage	22
Celery	21
Eggplant	21
Tomatoes	18
Onions	16
Beets	15
Pumpkin	12
Potatoes	11
Yams	8
Sweet Potatoes	6

GRAINS	%
Wheat germ	31
Rye	20
Wheat, hard red	17
Wild rice	16
Buckwheat	15
Oatmeal	15
Millet	12
Barley	11
Brown rice	8

FRUITS	%
Lemons	16
Honeydew melon	10
Cantaloupe	9
Strawberry	8
Orange	8
Blackberry	8
Cherry	8
Apricot	8
Grape	8
Watermelon	8
Tangerine	7
Papaya	6
Peach	6
Pear	5
Banana	5
Grapefruit	5
Pineapple	3
Apple	1

NUTS AND SEEDS	%
Pumpkin seeds	21
Sunflower seeds	17
Walnuts, black	13
Sesame seeds	13
Almonds	12
Cashews	12
Filberts	8

53

Data obtained from *Nutritive Value of American Foods in Common Units*, USDA Agriculture Handbook No. 456. Reprinted with author's permission, from *Diet for a New America* by John Robbins (Walpole, NH: Stillpoint Publishing).

The Miracle of Fasting*
Master Key to Internal Purification

If you do a complete water fast for 24 hours each week, soon you will be able to add more fresh fruit and vegetables to your diet. After a fast of 3 or more days, then you can include more foods that are in a high rate of vibration.

I faithfully fast for 24 hours every Monday and the first three days of each month. Wait until you experience this! You will greatly benefit from the inner cleansing and will love the pure, clean, healthy feeling you receive!

Fasting Cleanses, Renews and Rejuvenates

Our bodies have a natural self-cleansing and healing system for maintaining a healthy body and our "river of life" – our bloodstream. It's essential that we keep our entire bodily machinery from head to toes in perfect health and in good working order to maintain life!

Fasting is the best detoxifying method. It's also the most effective and safest way to increase elimination of waste buildups and enhance the body's miraculous self-healing and self-repairing process that keeps you healthy.

If you prepare for a fast by eating a cleansing diet for 1 to 2 days, this can greatly help the cleansing process. Fresh variety salads, fresh vegetables and fruits and their juices, as well as green drinks (alfalfa, barley, chlorophyll, chlorella, spirulina, wheatgrass, etc.) stimulate waste elimination. Fresh foods and juices can literally pick up dead matter from your body and carry it away.

Daily, even on most days during our fasts, we take 3,000 mg. of mixed vitamin C powder (C concentrate, acerola, rosehips and bioflavonoids) in liquids. This is a potent antioxidant and flushes out deadly free radicals that produce harmful effects, cancer, etc. Vitamin C also promotes collagen production for new healthy tissues and is especially important if you are detoxifying from prescription drugs or alcohol overload.

*For important fasting and cleansing information read the life-changing Bragg book, "The Miracle of Fasting." See back pages for booklist.

Fasting Removes Sludge from Your Pipes

A moderate, well planned distilled water fast (our favorite) or a diluted fresh juice (35% distilled water) fast for beginners can also cleanse your body of excess mucus, old fecal matter, trapped cellular, non-food wastes and help remove inorganic mineral deposits and sludge from your pipes and joints. (See pages 63-66 for juice fasting and combination juices, etc.)

Fasting works by self-digestion. During a fast your body intuitively will decompose and burn only substances and tissues that are damaged, diseased or unneeded, such as abscesses, tumors, excess fat deposits, excess water and congestive wastes. Even a relatively short fast (1 to 3 days) will accelerate elimination from your liver, kidneys, lungs, bloodstream and skin. Sometimes you will experience dramatic changes (cleansing and healing crises) as accumulated wastes are expelled. With your first fasts you may temporarily have headaches, fatigue, body odor, bad breath, coated tongue, mouth sores and even diarrhea as your body is cleaning house. Please be patient with your miracle body!

After a fast your body will begin to self-cleanse and healthfully rebalance! When you follow The Bragg Healthy Lifestyle, your weekly 24 hour fast removes toxins on a regular basis, so they don't accumulate. Your energy levels will amazingly begin to rise – physically, psychologically and mentally. Your creativity will begin to expand. You will feel like a different person – which you are – for now you are being cleansed, purified and reborn. It's an exciting and wonderful miracle!

Fasting Brings Remarkable Results

Professor A.E. Crews of Edinburgh University, who studied both worms and animals, said: *"Given appropriate and essential conditions, including proper care of the body, Eternal Youth can be a reality in living forms! It's possible, by repeated processes of fasting, to keep an earthworm alive twenty times longer than normal. This has also been proven with animals."* Something to think about that proves the life-extending merits of fasting!

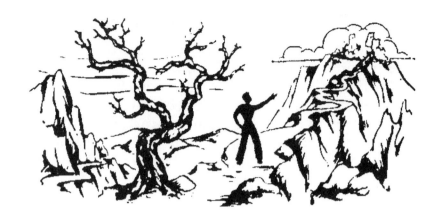

The Trail to Perfect Health

My father and I are very sincere about our fasting program. We know what it has done for us, for the members of our family, our friends, and thousands of Bragg health conscious students all over the world. So The Bragg Healthy Lifestyle calls for 4 longer fasts a year, along with a faithful weekly 24 or 36 hour fast. I always fast the first 3 days of every month and all day each Monday. Also, I usually take my longer, cleansing fasts at the beginning of each season.

Remember, it took time for the body to build up toxins, so it takes time to cleanse and unload them! Take your time! Be faithful to The Bragg Healthy Lifestyle. You will reap wonderful, priceless, long-lasting health benefits. Please read our book the *Miracle of Fasting* as it gives more details about the many benefits of fasting.

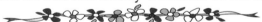

By relieving the body of the work of digesting foods, fasting allows the system to rid itself of toxins while facilitating healing. Fasting regularly gives your organs a rest and helps reverse the ageing process for a longer and healthier life.
– James F. Balch, M.D. Prescription for Nutritional Healing

Fasting clears away the thousand little things which quickly accumulate and clutter the body, mind and heart. It cuts through corrosion and renews our contract with God. – Paul C. Bragg

Actress Cloris Leachman is an ardent health follower who sparkles with health. She hates smoking, coffee, alcohol, sugar and meat. One of her solutions to health problems is to fast. "Fasting is simply wonderful. I can do practically anything. It is a miracle cure. It cured my asthma."

"Secret" of Health is Internal Cleanliness

What you want to strive for is a clean, toxicless body! Gradually include more organic, fresh fruit and raw vegetables in your diet. Have fresh fruit in the morning and a large raw, combination vegetable salad at noon. If you like, you may have some fresh fruit for dessert. Eat a yellow vegetable, such as a yam, sweet potato, yellow squash or carrots, and a green vegetable every day. Cook these vegetables by baking, steaming or wok (stir-fry) them. Always remember to save some raw vegetables for your cleansing garden variety salad.

With your main meal, at times you may have a more concentrated form of protein. My favorite, and the healthiest forms of protein, are vegetarian! If you insist on eating animal proteins, do so no more than 2 to 3 times a week. Your diet should include raw nuts and seeds (such as almonds, pecans, cashews, sunflower, pumpkin, sesame, etc.) and avocados. Enjoy beans, brown rice and legumes, soybeans and tofu as often as desired. By having a variety of God's natural foods you will enjoy a balanced diet and a healthier life!

You may use the natural, cold or expeller pressed oils, such as olive, flax, soy, safflower or sesame. Read labels carefully before buying products. I like to put virgin olive oil over my baked potatoes, instead of salt-free butter. Also, try a little olive oil over rice, lentils, beans and vegetables. Foods are extra delicious with a spray of Bragg Liquid Aminos, the perfect and delicious all-purpose health seasoning – now available in spray bottles at health food stores nationwide. Also, try a sprinkle of kelp seasoning or my favorite, nutritional brewer's yeast – the large flake variety tastes better.

The best way to eat potatoes is baked. I use a fast method of baking. Thoroughly scrub potato (either white, yam or sweet). Don't wrap or oil it. Bake in a 450° oven for 25 minutes. This converts the starch of the potato to a blood sugar. Be sure to eat the skin, too! Baked this fast way, it's crunchy and delicious. I don't

---

In regions where meat is scarce, cardiovascular disease is unknown.
– Time Magazine article

BENEFITS FROM THE JOYS OF FASTING

Fasting is easier than any diet. • Fasting is the quickest way to lose weight.
Fasting is adaptable to a busy life. • Fasting gives the body a physiological rest.
Fasting is used successfully in the treatment of many physical illnesses.
Fasting can yield weight losses of up to 10 pounds or more in the first week.
Fasting lowers & normalizes cholesterol and blood pressure levels.
Fasting is a calming experience, often relieving tension and insomnia.
Fasting improves dietary habits. • Fasting increases eating pleasure.
Fasting frequently induces feelings of euphoria, a natural *high*.
Fasting is a rejuvenator, slowing the ageing process.
Fasting is an energizer, not a debilitator. • Fasting aids the elimination process.
Fasting often results in a more vigorous sex life.
Fasting can eliminate or modify smoking, drug and drinking addictions.
Fasting is a regulator, educating the body to consume food only as needed.
Fasting saves time spent marketing, preparing and eating.
Fasting rids the body of toxins, giving it an "internal shower" & cleansing.
Fasting does not deprive the body of essential nutrients.
Fasting can be used to uncover the sources of food allergies.
Fasting is used effectively in schizophrenia treatment & other mental illnesses.
Fasting under proper supervision can be tolerated easily up to 4 weeks.
Fasting does not accumulate appetite; hunger "pangs" disappear in 1-2 days.
Fasting is routine for the animal kingdom.
Fasting has been a common practice since man's existence.
Fasting is a rite in all religions; the Bible alone has 74 references to it.
Fasting under proper conditions is absolutely safe.
Fasting is not starving, it's nature's cure that God has given us. – Patricia Bragg
— Allan Cott, M.D., *Fasting As A Way Of Life*

Spiritual Bible Reasons Why We Should Fast
For a Healthier, Happier, Longer Walk With Our Creator

3 John 2	Deut. 11:7-15,21	Luke 9:11	Matthew 9: 9-15
Gen. 6:3	Gal. 5:13-26	Mark 2:16-20	Neh. 9:1, 20-24
I Cor. 7:5	Isaiah 58	Matthew 4:1-4	Psalms 35:13
II Cor. 6	James 5:10-20	Matthew 6:6-18	Romans 16:16-20
Deut. 8:3	John 15	Matthew 7	Zachariah 8:1

Dear HEALTH FRIEND,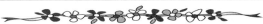

This gentle reminder explains the great benefits from *The Miracle of Fasting* that you will enjoy when starting on your weekly, 24 hour, Bragg Fasting Program for Super Health! It's a precious time of body-mind-soul cleansing and renewal.

On fast days I drink 8 to 10 glasses of distilled water, some with ACV. You may also have some herbal teas and if just starting try diluted fresh juices (add ⅓ distilled water). Every day, even some fast days, add 1 tbsp. of this mixture (½ oat bran and ½ psyllium husk powder) to liquids once daily. It's an extra cleanser and helps normalize weight, cholesterol and blood pressure and helps promote healthy elimination. Fasting is the oldest, most effective healing method known to man. Fasting offers great, miraculous blessings from Mother Nature and our Creator. It begins the self-cleansing of the inner-body workings so we can promote our own self-healing.

My father and I wrote the book *The Miracle of Fasting* to share with you the health miracles it can perform in your daily life. It's all so worthwhile to do and it's an important part of The Bragg Healthy Lifestyle.

With Love, *Patricia*

Paul Bragg's work on fasting and water is one of the great contributions to Healing Wisdom and the Natural Health Movement in the world today.
– Gabriel Cousens, M.D., Author, *Conscious Eating & Spiritual Nutrition*

believe in microwaves that destroy food cells, as irradiation also does. A fair priced, safer alternative is the convection oven. It's almost as fast as the deadly microwave and can be built in or placed on your kitchen countertop.

We never use table salt – it should have no place in your diet! Salt is an inorganic substance and only causes problems in the body! Organic sodium found naturally in "live" foods is best. Read labels and don't buy products that add salt!

Avoid Refined, Processed, Unhealthy Foods!

Eliminate refined, white flour products and white sugar products entirely. Eat no mushy, dead, refined cereals or those dry commercial cereals, for they are in a low rate of vibration, despite having been enriched with chemically produced vitamins and minerals. (Health Food Stores carry natural organic cereals, if you desire a whole grain cereal.)

Avoid these foods: Fried, salted, refined, preserved and chemicalized foods; coffee, China tea, cola and alcohol drinks; sugared, salted juices; overcooked, oversalted vegetables and salted, creamed or flour-thickened soups. Read page 86 for a complete foods-to-avoid list.

(59)

You now know the foods to avoid: Refined, unhealthy foods high in fat, salt and sugar; meat and dairy products; and chemicalized and sugared foods and beverages.

You now know the foods you can eat: Fresh fruits (organically grown is always best to buy or grow yourself); fresh juices; raw variety salads; fresh vegetables steamed, baked or wokked; vegetable proteins; beans, legumes, tofu, nuts, seeds, etc. If you really want animal and fish proteins, limit them to twice weekly. Occasionally, eat nothing but fruits or fruits and raw vegetables for 1 or 2 days a week. Remember, vegetarians are the healthiest among Americans! Research proves this!

Use your imagination to plan enjoyable, live food meals that are in a high rate of vibration. Above all, eat simply. Avoid eating too many mixtures of food. Don't overeat. Be moderate in all things for the best of health.

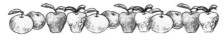

Who is strong? He that can conquer his bad habits. – Ben Franklin

Eat only when you are really hungry, not because it is mealtime. Earn your food by activity, vigorous exercise and deep breathing. You will see how much more you enjoy your food when you deserve and earn it!

The Miracle Powers of Fruits

Always keep in mind that the most perfect food for man is fresh, ripe fruits. Mother Nature, in her unique way, brings together in her fruits a marvelous balance. The fruits are living combinations of vital principles, in high rates of vibration, bio-magnetized, to release the living building blocks so necessary to maintain life.

Tinted by basking in the rays of the vitalizing sun, taking in draughts of magnetized air, drawing into itself vital minerals through its roots in the earth, delicious, organic fruits are God's perfect creations!

Man can get all the chemicals of an apple out of a chemist's dish, but he cannot construct an apple! Man may analyze all the minerals of a cherry, but he does not even know what makes it red. He may take apart and try to reconstruct a grape, and find that the grape supports life, but the broken down chemicals do not!

Fruits contain bioelectric principles that give electric sparks of life! Organic fruits are the most perfect foods from Mother Nature and God. Fruits will support life indefinitely to a superior degree when a body is cleansed and living in a natural environment. Ask your grocer to stock organically grown produce – it's the healthiest!

Who has not had his mouth water when seeing a luscious dish of delicious, ripe fruit before him - for instance some yellow pears with a dash of pink or a beautiful bunch of tapering grapes, green, red or blue? The sight of fruits and the taste of them, more so, bring an abundant secretion of digestive juices, for fruits are the most natural foods. I can say without reserve that fruits are designed beautifully for our digestive tracts.

A favor or kindness is best when given freely, without any motive, strings or reminders.

A reminder: What's on the plate becomes what's on the chair.

I have seen a sick person turn down all other foods for some freshly squeezed orange juice. His sick body craved the nutrients in juicy oranges. I have seen children torn with fever ask for fruit juice. Why didn't they ask for a hot dog? Mother Nature's guidance was in force.

But diets that consist solely of fruits are impractical for the average American, although they would be splendid for short periods in a tropical climate. While we have come so far from our natural state that we can't maintain an efficient lifestyle as 100% fruitarians, we still need to eat plenty of fresh fruits! One of the many reasons I love Hawaii are the luscious tropical fruits! Plan a Hawaiian vacation soon and enjoy the free Bragg Exercise Class at Waikiki Beach in Honolulu. It's going strong and thousands of Bragg followers from around the world annually visit the class. Info on page iii.

I especially recommend ripe bananas. Bananas are not a fattening fruit, as is commonly supposed. They are 70% water and are extremely high in potassium. Organic apples of all kinds make excellent eating, as do pears and grapes. In the fall, winter and spring, eat organically grown dates, sun-dried figs, raisins and apricots along with fresh fruits. When you eat fruits, see how light and wonderful you feel and look!

Avocado is Mother Nature's Miracle Food

The avocado tree is strong and insects don't bother it. It requires no spraying with poisonous chemicals. The avocado has a perfect balance – high vibration of life-giving nutrients. It has an unsaturated fat which the body can handle perfectly and more potassium than bananas! I eat avocados from my Santa Barbara ranch three to four times a week. I mash the avocado, add fresh minced garlic and a dash of olive oil and Bragg Liquid Aminos. I dip slices of tomato, celery, carrot, turnip, cabbage, radish, cucumber, red and green bell pepper and lettuce leaves into this "guacamole" for a delicious healthy lunch.

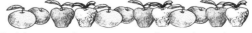

Nothing transforms a person faster than changing from a negative to a positive attitude. – Paul C. Bragg

Foods in a High Vibration
Contain Life-Giving Substance

When you eat only foods that are in a high vibration, your body performs and operates by God's Universal Law and becomes a self-starting, self-governing, self-generating instrument! I want you to live by Mother Nature's and God's Laws so your body will be a fine working instrument for you at every age. If you have the desire to retain the vivacity, vitality, energy and enthusiasm of youth and the desire to turn back the clock of Father Time, when your body is bent, your eyes are dimmed and your gait is halting at an age when you should be buoyant with the spirit of youth, then I say:

"There is but one way to live and that is Mother Nature's and God's Healthy Way!"

With Your Hands You Prepare Either Health or Sickness – It's Up to You

They who provide the food for the world, decide the health of the world. A vast multitude of the human race are slaughtered by incompetent cookery. Though you may have taken lessons in music, painting or astronomy, you are not well-educated unless you have taken lessons in preparing healthy meals. You can either prepare health or sickness with your two hands. Healthy nutritional planning produces good performance.

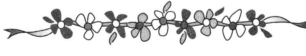

Ponce de Leon

Searched for the "Fountain of Youth."
If he had only known
It's within us . . .
Created by food we eat!
Food can make or
break your health!

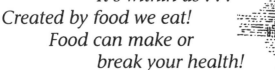

Juice Fast – Introduction to Water Fast

Fasting has been rediscovered through juice fasting — as a simple, easy means of cleansing and restoring health and vitality. To fast (abstain from food) comes from the Old English word fasten or to hold firm. It's a means to commit oneself to the task of finding inner strength through body, mind and soul cleansing. Throughout history the world's greatest philosophers and sages, including Socrates, Plato, Buddha and Gandhi, have enjoyed fasting and preached its benefits.

Juice bars are springing up everywhere and juice fasting has become "in" with the theatrical crowd in Hollywood, New York and in London. The number of Stars who believe in the power and effectiveness of juice and water fasting is growing. A partial list includes: Steven Spielberg, Barbra Streisand, Kim Basinger, Alec Baldwin, Daryl Hannah, Donna Karan, Christie Brinkley and Cloris Leachman. They say fasting helps balance their lives physically, mentally and emotionally.

Although a pure water fast is best, an introductory liquid juice fast can offer people an ideal opportunity to give their intestinal systems a restful, cleansing relief from the commercial high fat, high sugar, high salt and high protein fast foods too many Americans exist on.

Organic, raw, live fruit and vegetable juices can be purchased fresh from many Health Food Stores. You can also prepare these healthy juices yourself using a good home juicer. When juice fasting, it's then best to dilute juice with ⅓ distilled water. This list gives you many combination ideas. With vegetable and tomato combinations try adding a dash of Bragg Liquid Aminos, herbs or, on non-fast days, even some green powder (alfalfa, barley, chlorella, spirulina, etc.) to create a delicious, nutritious powerful health drink. When using herbs in these drinks, use 1 to 2 fresh leaves or a pinch of dried herbs. A pinch of dulse (seaweed) rich in protein, iodine and iron – is delicious with vegetable juices.

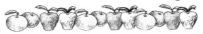

Fasting is the greatest remedy – the physician within!
– Paracelsus, 15th century physician
who established the role of chemistry in medicine

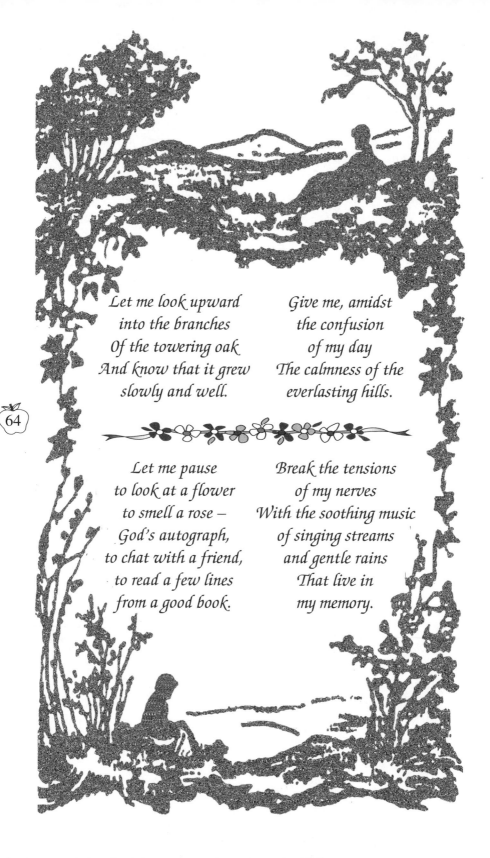

Let me look upward
into the branches
Of the towering oak
And know that it grew
slowly and well.

Give me, amidst
the confusion
of my day
The calmness of the
everlasting hills.

Let me pause
to look at a flower
to smell a rose —
God's autograph,
to chat with a friend,
to read a few lines
from a good book.

Break the tensions
of my nerves
With the soothing music
of singing streams
and gentle rains
That live in
my memory.

Here are Some Powerful Juice Combinations:

1. Beet, celery, alfalfa sprouts
2. Cabbage, celery and apple
3. Cabbage, cucumber, celery, tomato, spinach and basil
4. Tomato, carrot and mint
5. Carrot, celery, watercress, garlic and wheatgrass
6. Grapefruit, orange and lemon
7. Beet, parsley, celery, carrot, mustard greens, garlic
8. Beet, celery, dulse and carrot
9. Cucumber, carrot and parsley
10. Watercress, cucumber, garlic
11. Asparagus, carrot, and mint
12. Carrot, celery, parsley, onion, cabbage and sweet basil
13. Carrot and coconut milk
14. Carrot, broccoli, lemon, cayenne
15. Carrot, cauliflower, rosemary
16. Apple, carrot, radish, ginger
17. Apple, pineapple and mint
18. Apple, papaya and grapes
19. Papaya, cranberries and apple
20. Leafy greens, broccoli, apple
21. Grape, cherry and apple
22. Watermelon (include seeds)

Juicing has come a long way since Paul C. Bragg imported the first hand operated vegetable-fruit juicer from Germany and introduced juice therapy to America. Before this, juice was pressed by hand using cheesecloth. Juices are now considered an ideal health beverage around the world!

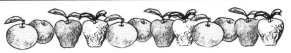

Through our actions and deeds, rather than promises,
let us display the essence of love – perfect harmony in motion!
– Philip Glyn, Welsh Poet

Kindness should be a frame of mind in which we are alert
to every chance to do, to give, to share and to cheer.

Little deeds of kindness, little words of love,
Help to make earth happy, like the Heaven above.
– Julia A. F. Carney

Kindness comes in all sizes.
Sometimes it is only
A little thing we give –
A trifle, a smile, a piece of fruit,
A hug, and a kind word.
If it is given willingly,
The kindness is doubled. – Syrus

Liquefied and Fresh Juiced Foods

The juicer, food processor and blender are great for preparing foods for gentle or bland diets and baby foods. Fibers of fresh fruits and vegetables juiced can be tolerated on most gentle diets. Any raw or cooked fruit or vegetable can be liquefied and added to non-dairy Rice Dream, nut or soy milks or broth or soups. Live, fresh juices super charge your body's health power! You may fortify your liquid meal with barley green, alfalfa, chlorella or spirulina powder for extra nutrition.

The Bragg Healthy Lifestyle Promotes Super Health & Longevity

The Bragg Healthy Lifestyle consists of eating a diet of 60% to 70% fresh, live, organically grown foods; raw vegetables, salads, fresh fruits and juices; sprouts, raw seeds and nuts; all-natural 100% whole-grain breads, pastas, cereals and nutritious beans and legumes. These are the no cholesterol, no fat, no salt, "live foods" which combine to make up the body fuel that creates healthy, lively people that want to exercise and be fit. This healthy diet also creates energy. This is the reason people become revitalized and reborn into a fresh new life filled with joy, health, vitality, youthfulness and longevity! There are millions of healthy Bragg followers around the world proving that this lifestyle works!

Pure Water Is Important for Health

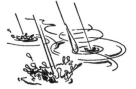

To the days of the aged it addeth length;
To the might of the strong it addeth strength;
It freshens the heart, it brings the sight;
'Tis like drinking a goblet of morning light.

The body is 70% water and pure, steam-distilled (chemical-free) water is important for total health. You should drink 7-9 glasses of water a day. Read our revealing book, Water – The Shocking Truth for more needed information on the importance of pure water.

Drinking 8 glasses daily of pure distilled water
cleanses and recharges the human batteries! – Paul C. Bragg

Distilled Water is Safest and Best for Health

Pure distilled water is vitally important in following The Bragg Healthy Lifestyle. Water is the key to all body functions including: digestion, assimilation, elimination and circulation, and to bones and joints, muscles, nerves, glands and senses. The right kind of water is one of your best natural protections against all kinds of diseases and infections. It's a vital factor in all body fluids, tissues, cells, lymph, blood and all glandular secretions. Water holds all nutritive factors in solution, as well as toxins and body wastes, and acts as the main transportation medium throughout the body, for both nutrition and cleansing purposes.

Since your body is about 70% water, the blood and lymphatic system over 90% water, it's essential for your health you consistently drink only pure water that's not saturated with contaminants, inorganic minerals and toxins. This water will transport vital nutrients to cells and waste from cells more efficiently. This allows the body to function correctly and stay healthier!

ORGANIC MINERALS. Your minerals must come from an organic source, from something living or that has lived. Humans do not have the same chemistry as plants. Only the living plant has the ability to extract inorganic minerals from the earth and convert them to organic minerals for your body to absorb and utilize.

INORGANIC MINERALS. Inorganic minerals and toxic chemicals in water can create these problems:

- Clog and harden the veins, capillaries and arteries.
- Cause arthritis, bone spurs and painful calcified formations in the joints.
- Harden the liver.
- Cause kidney and gallstones.
- Inorganic minerals and the toxic chemicals in water clog the arteries and small capillaries that are needed to feed and nourish your brain with oxygenated blood; the result is loss of memory and gradual senility and strokes.

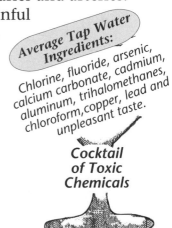

Average Tap Water Ingredients:

Chlorine, fluoride, arsenic, calcium carbonate, cadmium, aluminum, trihalomethanes, chloroform, copper, lead and unpleasant taste.

Cocktail of Toxic Chemicals

Skin Absorbs Water, Toxins and All!

*Compared with its absorption through the respiratory system, skin absorption could be the major route of penetration into the body. Skin penetration rates have been found to be remarkably high, and the outer layer of skin is a less effective barrier to penetration than traditionally assumed. Factors affecting absorption are:

Hydration: The more hydrated the skin, the greater the absorption. If the skin is hydrated by perspiration or immersion in water or if the contaminant compounds are in solution, penetration is enhanced.

Temperature: Increased skin or water temperature will enhance skin absorption capacity proportionately. During swimming and bathing, it may be expected that greater hydration of skin surfaces will take place.

Skin Condition: Any insult (i.e. sunburn) or injury (i.e. cuts, wounds, abrasions) to the skin will lower its ability to act as a barrier against foreign substances. A history of skin disease such as psoriasis or eczema acts to lower the natural barrier of the outer skin layer, as do rashes, dermatitis, or any chronic skin condition.

Regional Variability: Skin absorption rates vary with the different regions of the body. Underestimated is the case of whole body immersion during swimming or bathing. The epidermis of the hand represents a relatively greater barrier to penetration than many other parts of the body, including the scalp, forehead, abdomen, area in and around the ears, underarms and genital area. Penetration through the genital area is estimated to be 100% but only 8.6% for the forearm.

Other Routes of Entry: Other routes of absorption include oral, nasal, cheeks and mouth cavity, and eye and ear areas. These routes have been underestimated in their ability to absorb contaminants during immersion in water. Inhalation serves as yet another route. In the case of swimming or bathing, the volatilized chemicals are likely to gather near the surface of the water and are readily inhalable. In addition, some may be swallowed.

— * From *the American Journal of Public Health*

You Get More Toxic Exposure from Taking a Shower Than From Drinking the Same Water!

*Two of the very highly volatile and toxic chemicals, trichloroethylene and chloroform have been proven as toxic contaminants found in most municipal drinking-water supplies. The great National Academy of Sciences recently has estimated that 200 to 1,000 people die in the United States

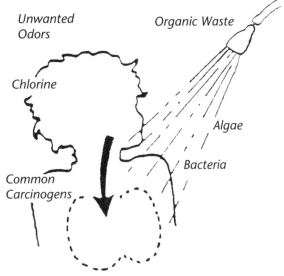

Unwanted Odors

Organic Waste

Chlorine

Algae

Bacteria

Common Carcinogens

each year from the cancers caused largely by ingesting water pollutants from inhalation as air pollutants in the home. Inhalation exposure to water pollutants has largely been ignored. Data indicates that hot showers can liberate about 50% of the chloroform and 80% of the trichloroethylene into the air.

Tests show that your body can absorb more chlorine as a result of a 10-minute shower than if you drank 8 glasses of the same water. How can that be? A warm shower opens up your pores, causing your skin to act like a sponge. As a result, you not only inhale the chlorine vapors, you absorb them through your skin, directly into your bloodstream – at a rate that's up to 6 times higher than drinking it.

In terms of cumulative damage to your health, showering in chlorinated water is one of the most dangerous risks you take daily. Short-term risks include: eyes, sinus, throat, skin and lung irritation. Long-term risks include: excessive free radical formation (that ages you faster!), higher vulnerability to genetic mutation and cancer development, difficulty metabolizing cholesterol which can cause hardened arteries. – * From Science News

Five Hidden Dangers in Your Shower:

• **Chlorine:** Added to all municipal water supplies, this disinfectant hardens arteries, destroys proteins in the body, irritates skin and sinus conditions and aggravates any asthma, allergies and respiratory problems.

• **Chloroform:** This powerful by-product of chlorination causes excessive free radical formation (a cause of accelerated ageing!), normal cells to mutate and cholesterol to form. It's a known carcinogen!

• **DCA (Dichloroacedic acid):** This chlorine by-product alters cholesterol metabolism and has been shown to cause liver cancer in lab animals.

• **MX (another chlorinated acid):** Another by-product of chlorination, MX is known to cause genetic mutations that can lead to cancer growth and has been found in all chlorinated water for which it was tested.

• **Proven cause of bladder and rectal cancer:** Research proved that chlorinated water is the direct cause of 9% of all US bladder cancers and 15% of all rectal cancers.

Showers, Toxic Chemicals & Chlorine

Skin absorption of toxic contaminants has been underestimated and ingestion may not constitute the sole or even primary route of exposure.
– Dr. Halina Brown, *American Journal of Public Health*

Taking long hot showers is a health risk, according to the latest research. Showers – and to a lesser extent baths – lead to a greater exposure to toxic chemicals contained in water supplies than does drinking the water. These toxic chemicals evaporate out of the water and are inhaled. They can also spread through the house and be inhaled by others. People receive 6 to 100 times more chemicals by breathing the air around showers and baths than they would by drinking the water.
– Ian Anderson, *New Scientist*

A professor of Water Chemistry at the University of Pittsburgh claims that exposure to vaporized chemicals in the water supplies through showering, bathing, and inhalation is 100 times greater than through drinking the water. – *The Nader Report – Troubled Waters on Tap*

Chlorine is the greatest crippler and killer of modern times. While it prevented epidemics of one disease, it was creating another. Twenty years after the start of chlorinating our drinking water in 1904, the present epidemic of heart trouble, cancer and senility began.
– Dr. Joseph Price, *Coronaries/Cholesterol/Chlorine*

Don't Gamble With Your Health – Use a Shower Filter

The most effective method of removing hazards from your shower is the quick and easy installation of a filter on your shower arm. The filter we found to be the best removes chlorine, lead, mercury, iron, chlorine by-products, arsenic, hydrogen sulfide, and many other unseen contaminants, such as bacteria, fungi, dirt and sediments. It has a 12-18 month filter life-span. The filter is easily cleaned by backwashing every 2-3 months and is replaceable. For info on the best shower filter call 800-446-1990. I have been using this filter for over 3 years and am really thankful for my chlorine-free showers!

Start enjoying safe, chlorine-free showers right away. It's essential to reducing your risk of heart disease and cancer and to ease the strain from your immune system. And you may even get rid of long-standing conditions – from sinus and respiratory problems to dry, itchy skin.

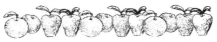

Urgent Health Alert!

Thousands of gallons of the potentially deadly gas additive methyl tertiary butyl ether – or MTBE – are leaking every day into our precious water supplies from underground storage tanks across the United States! This chemical, which is purported to reduce car emissions and is mandated by Federal law is suspected of causing a wide range of diseases including asthma, nosebleeds and cancer. It has even appeared in the pristine water of Lake Tahoe!
Act now! *Call or write your government representatives today! Join your local chapter of an action group (like OxyBusters, Greenpeace or the Sierra Club) before this 3 billion dollar a year rip off pollutes our water forever.*

Perfect health is above gold; a sound body before riches. – Solomon

---

You can change the quality of your health by detoxifying your body.
Start Your Bragg Healthy Lifestyle today!

Comparison of Water Treatment Methods

POLLUTANT	Filter Sediment	Filter Carbon	Deionization	Reverse Osmosis	Steam Distillation
Arsenic	○	○	●	●	●
Bacteria	○	○	○	◐	●
Cadmium	○	○	●	●	●
Calcium	○	○	●	●	●
Chlorides	○	○	●	●	●
Chlorine	○	●	○	●[1]	●[1]
Cryptosporidium	○	○	○	●	●
Detergents	○	◐	●	●	●
Fluorides	○	○	●	●	●
Lead	○	○	●	●	●
Magnesium	○	○	●	●	●
Nitrate	○	○	◐	◐	●
Organics	○	●	○	●[1]	●[1]
Pesticides	○	●	○	●[1]	●[1]
Phosphates	○	○	●	●	●
Radon	○	○	●	●	●
Sediment	●	◐	●	●	●
Sodium	○	○	●	●	●
Sulfates	○	◐	●	●	●
Viruses	○	○	○	○	●

○ Ineffective or No Reduction   ◐ Significant Reduction   ● Complete or Significant Reduction

1 – A Carbon Filter Needed (The best home distillers have carbon filters.)

72

For more info on water distillers for your home & shower head filters
to remove harmful chemicals from your shower water call 800-446-1990.

The kind of water you drink can make or break you – your body is 70% water.

Exercise is Vital for Health and Longevity

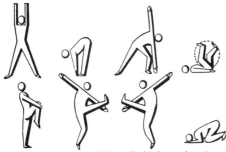

Stretch, bend, lift, roll, kick and twist

To ensure youthful arteries, exercise is essential! If you wish to live and enjoy a long, healthy life it's necessary to build up your cardio-vascular endurance and to follow a program designed to keep your arteries unclogged, soft, agile and healthy. The first step is to get more oxygen into the body which will help dissolve the encrustations that have formed in the arteries. Any physical activity that injects more oxygen is going to help extend your life!

Enjoy a Tireless – Ageless – Painless Body With The Bragg Healthy Lifestyle

Don't despair in your golden years – enjoy them! Paul C. Bragg, my dad, said life's second half is the best and can be the most fruitful years. Linus Pauling, Grandma Moses and the amazing Mother Teresa, have all proven that! Three famous men –Conrad Hilton, J.C. Penney and foot Dr. Scholl were all Bragg health followers and they lived strong, productive, active lives to almost 100. Countless others worldwide have lived long, healthy lives following The Bragg Healthy Lifestyle.

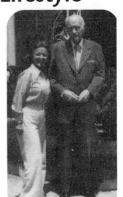

73

Conrad Hilton thanked the Braggs for his long healthy life.

We teach you how to forget calendar years and to regain not only a youthful spirit, but much of the vigor of your youth. It's your duty to yourself to start to live The Bragg Healthy Lifestyle today – don't procrastinate!

Square your shoulders and look life straight in the face. Keep premature ageing out of your body by following The Bragg Healthy Lifestyle Blueprint. You must eat foods that have a high rate of vibration (an abundance of raw, organic fruits and vegetables) and do a water fast one day a week.

Also, do some Bragg Super Power Deep Breathing exercises, get 8 hours of restful sleep at night and keep your body relaxed. Don't let anything rob you of your emotional and nervous energy and precious vital force. Do read our book *Build Powerful Nerve Force*.

Your body is being made anew every day! Premature ageing and senility result from toxic debris that accumulates when you live an unhealthy lifestyle. Eat right, exercise for good circulation throughout your body, and there will be little or no buildup of toxins that will clog and prematurely age your body.

Cultivate and hold onto the spirit of youth *and it will be yours!* You can feel and look younger! Keep your spine straight to maintain high energy level. Daily do The Bragg Posture Exercise on page 80. Follow The Bragg Healthy Lifestyle and miracles will follow!

If you are already in the clutches of premature ageing, begin now to fight for the return of youth. Work to restore this priceless possession! You can do it! Train your body as you would that of a race horse. Follow these clear, definite instructions and you will gain strength, virility, energy, vivacity and enthusiasm! Make your life a daily enjoyment of the most precious of all earthly gifts – the power and joys of youthful, healthful living. Men and women can be young at 60, 70, 80 and even 90! Some have retained the spirit of youth beyond the century mark, like the Hunzas of Kashmir and Georgians of Russia are still doing!

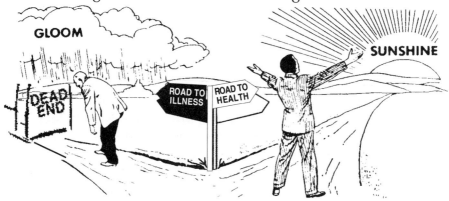

The choice of which road to take is up to the individual. He alone can decide whether he wants to reach a dead end or live a healthy lifestyle for a long, healthy, happy, active life. – Paul C. Bragg

Health Suggestions for Your Daily Program

Those of you who live the incomplete life, and give up the precious qualities of human existence for dietary excesses or for the pleasures of luxury and idleness, are selling your birthright for a mess of pottage!

Wake up to the possibilities within your reach! Rejuvenate your body. Make your mind keen and capable. Obey the laws of Mother Nature and God and you will see results that you now scarcely dare to dream!

Be sure that you sleep in a thoroughly ventilated, uncluttered, dust-free room, so you get a large amount of clean oxygen while sleeping. I know it's often difficult to keep dust collectors (knick-knacks, etc.) out of your home. We recently had to unclutter some areas due to dust mites. It's best to vacuum carpets often, using a hepa filter or a micro-liner bag. Put pillows and mattresses (dust mites' haven) in protective closed covers. Make sure your mattress is firm and flat. Sleep spread-out to allow for good circulation. It's best not to sleep in a cramped position or sleep on your arms.

Oxygen – The Invisible Staff of Life

Oxygen is the life of the blood, and blood is the life of the body! A person weighing about 150 pounds contains about 88 pounds of oxygen. Oxygen is the most important element in the body. It is colorless, odorless and tasteless. Its main function is purification. Lack of oxygen in the body can lead to serious consequences. The majority of people are oxygen starved because they are shallow breathers.*

To have a youthful, vital life, we need fresh, unpolluted air in abundance, pure distilled water and plenty of fresh organic vegetables and fruits. Remember, oxygen is an unquestionable source of indispensable energy necessary for higher vital activity in the human organism! It ensures elimination, reconstruction and regeneration within the vital factors and metabolic activities of the entire physical body.

*Read the Bragg book, *"Super Power Breathing for Super Energy,"* for amazing, easy-to-do breathing exercises that bring results!

Through the lung functioning, oxygen is absorbed and assimilated into the bloodstream, bringing with it other unknown factors from the atmosphere.

Plants, through their roots, absorb all the vital elements in the soil necessary for their life. If we cut or damage their roots, they die! Man's roots are his lungs. Smokers are killing their lungs and the lungs of all those around them! Try never to be around secondhand smoke – it's even more deadly!

We can only breathe adequately with sufficient physical movement. With the proper movements we are motivated to obtain the full elixir of life which is the breath of air. The stronger and more vigorous our movements, the more air we need and the deeper we breathe.

The oxygen in the air that we breathe dissolves and eliminates waste and builds the continuum of our cellular structure, thus maintaining our body to the highest degree possible! Each breath should detoxify and regenerate our vital forces. But this rejuvenation process must be supplemented by following The Bragg Healthy Lifestyle. I want it definitely understood that both exercise and conscious deep breathing must be fortified with proper healthy nutrition to prevent the degenerative process of the cells.

This explains why there is a physical decline in top athletes in their late 20s who haven't consumed a correct nutritionally, balanced diet. The average athlete reaches a peak at about 27 and then, sadly, begins to decline. I know this to be true, as my father was an active athlete for over 80 years and we saw the finest athletes reach their peak and then slowly decline, with many of them dying way too young.

Other factors affecting breathing: Our thoughts and emotions interfere with our breathing. That's why, if we have a headache or some other sudden symptom, a few minutes of deep breathing exercises in the open air will help us detoxify and reestablish our internal balance.

After years of asthma, within a month I could breath almost normally for the first time in my life. Fasting is a miracle and I thank Paul Bragg for the Miracle of Fasting *book that showed me the importance of eating healthy and fasting! –Paul Wenner, Creator Gardenburger, author of Garden Cuisine*

To Rest is to Rust and Rust is Destruction!

Upon waking in the morning, stretch your legs, arms and body as you do when yawning. Continue this stretching process until you feel that every muscle has been properly and fully awakened. Good circulation and elimination are the master keys to good health! That is the reason it is important to stretch and exercise your body. Don't restrict your exercises to the morning. Make some time for them during the day to keep your circulation strong throughout your cardiovascular system during all your waking hours. Don't sit longer than one hour at a time. Do some stretching and deep breathing exercises. Get up and move around. Don't sit in a car for more than an hour. Stop the car and get out and stretch. Exercise your legs and body. See page 73.

Exercises Will Help Keep You More Healthy, Youthful, Flexible and Fit

You must fight off stiffness if you want the body to feel youthful. Most prematurely old people find it impossible to straighten their spines or continually maintain good posture. Why? Because their bodies have become stiff and rigid through lack of exercise and use.

It is no wonder that men and women become prematurely old, settle down and get crusty and stiff-necked. They don't do exercises that move their spinal joints! If you have already begun to acquire this stiffness, take warning now and reverse old age habits!

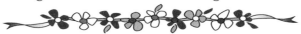

Give us Lord, a bit of sun,
A bit of work and a bit of fun.
Give us, in all struggle and sputter,
Our daily whole grain bread and food.
Give us health, our keep to make
And a bit to spare for others' sake.
Give us too, a bit of song
And a tale and a book, to help us along.
Give us Lord, a chance to be
Our goodly best for ourselves and others
Until men learn to live as brothers.

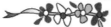 An Old English Prayer

Keep Spine Flexible and Youthful

Go to work on yourself! One of the main keys to looking 10 years younger is to keep your spine active, so strive for flexibility and elasticity in every part of your body, especially your spine! Also, remember to stand, walk and sit tall because all youthful-looking people have good posture.

The spine is a marvelous instrument as well as the central support of the whole body. It is made up of a flexible column of squarish bones that are joined together with rubbery puffs called discs. This wonderful piece of equipment stores its own lubrication in little sacs at the joints. The spine was designed for action! Keep it loose and supple, and your whole body will move with grace, ease and youthfulness. Read the Bragg *Fitness Spine Motion* Book for the Bragg Simple Spine Exercises to help keep your spine and you flexible and youthful.

Your Waistline is Your Life-Line, Date-Line and Health-Line!

Get a tape measure and measure your waist. Write down the measurement. If you consciously pursue vigorous abdominal and postural exercises combined with correct eating and a weekly 24 hour fast (and later on, 3 to 7 day fasts), in a short time you'll see a more trim and youthful waistline. Trim waistlines can make people appear years younger. Now, let's get yours down to where it should be, if it has grown too big and fat. It's a trim, lean horse for the long race of life! I'm sure we all want longevity! Studies show the bigger the waistline – the shorter the lifespan. Living The Bragg Healthy Lifestyle is so wonderful. Life and each day is a precious gift to enjoy, treasure and guard.

People abuse their abdomens abominably! You cannot eat dead, empty-calorie foods and tell yourself that a tiny snack here and there won't show! You are completely wrong! Dead, devitalized foods create toxic poisons inside your body and this all helps to add flabby unhealthy fat and inches to your abdomen.

The body is self-cleansing, self-correcting and self-healing when you give it a chance! – Patricia Bragg

Large Waistlines Lead to Shorter Lifespans

Do not overeat even healthy foods, for your body only needs enough food (fuel) to maintain health and energy. People become overweight because they have over-fueled into their bodies. Studies show large waistlines produce shorter lifespans.

You are not getting away with this kind of cheating, you are just cheating (hurting) yourself! Bear in mind that as we live longer, the internal abdominal structure and stomach muscles relax more. This is called visceroptosis, or droopy tummy. It's a common condition among older people who don't exercise their waist muscles. It can be a contributing cause of constipation, sluggish liver and even hernias.

When the abdominal wall becomes lazy and the consequent droop is compounded by fatty layers of flab, trouble starts inside the abdomen. By the time most people reach 40, they have a prolapsed abdomen. Become a people watcher and you will notice that what I'm saying is true! Some need a surgical tummy-tuck (which removes excess flab) to give them a flat stomach. So, don't let your abdominal muscles droop! Make every effort to recapture firmness. It's amazing how quickly muscles respond to exercises and good posture.

Maintain Youthful Posture for Super-Health

There is a fundamental relationship between good posture and youth on the one hand and between bent posture and age on the other! To maintain the posture of youth actually means to maintain youth itself, because of the basic relationship between the healthy, normal spine and bodily vigor: the condition that signifies youth, irrespective of how many years one has lived.

The most easily recognized sign of premature ageing is the forward bending of the spine, combined with the "rounded shoulders" that accompany it. Prematurely old people often exhibit this condition to an extreme degree, almost bending over double. Even school children sometimes display early signs of premature ageing . . .

All pleasures are tasteless without health. – Fred Van Amburgh

poor posture, stooped, rounded shoulders, and sunken-in chests! On the other hand, people of advanced years, by simply straightening their spines and walking erect, appear 10 to 30 years younger than they really are. Look around you and start noticing postures and you will see what I mean!

One's entire life must be a constant fight to maintain the correct, erect position, for this gives your heart and internal organs room to operate more efficiently. Remember, the spine is the fundamental structure of the body. Along with the brain, the spine constitutes the center of the nervous system. All other parts of the body are, so to speak, appendages of the spine. Keep that spinal column straight, keep it flexible and youthful! Good health and longevity depend on a healthy, erect body. Never cross your legs – sit tall with both feet on floor. Stretch up your spine to sit, stand and walk tall. Look at your posture in the mirror. See where you are on the posture chart – perfect, fair or poor? Start improving from today on!

Bragg Posture Exercise Gives Youthfulness

Before a mirror, stand up, feet 8" apart, stretch up spine. Tighten buttocks and suck in stomach muscles, lift up rib cage, put chest out, shoulders back, and chin up slightly. Line body up straight (nose plumbline straight to belly button), drop hands to sides and swing arms to normalize your posture. Do this posture exercise daily and miraculous changes will happen! You are retraining and strengthening your muscles to stand straight for health and youthfulness. Remember when you slump, you also cramp your precious machinery. This posture exercise will retrain your frame to sit, stand and walk tall for supreme health and longevity!

Where there is love, there is life. – Gandhi

Physical activity need not be strenuous to achieve health benefits.
– U.S. Surgeon General's Report, 1997

A strong body makes the mind strong. – Thomas Jefferson, 3rd U.S. President

----

I like the laughter that opens the lips and the heart, that
shows at the same time the pearls and the soul. – Victor Hugo

POSTURE CHART

	PERFECT	FAIR	POOR
HEAD			
SHOULDERS			
SPINE			
HIPS			
ANKLES			
NECK			
UPPER BACK			
TRUNK			
ABDOMEN			
LOWER BACK			

81

Your posture carries you through life from your head to your feet. This is your human vehicle and you are truly a miracle! Cherish, respect and always protect it by living The Bragg Healthy Lifestyle. – Patricia Bragg

Prevention is always preferable to cure!

Stop Dying – Start Living

The Bible tells us that . . .

The kingdom of Heaven is within us.

I thoroughly believe this statement! We can make this body we live in either a kingdom of heaven on earth or we can make it a torture chamber. It's all up to you!

After childhood, the kind of body you live in is strictly up to you! I cannot live your life for you! Nor can anyone else! You are a mature adult, and you must face the realities of life. I am sure you have the willpower and desire to follow The Bragg Healthy Lifestyle, so start on the road to Higher Health today!

This is the Bragg Master Blueprint to greater physical perfection because it works with the Laws of God and Mother Nature, and they make no compromises! You either follow them or they break you! You cannot break a natural law or a God law, for it only breaks you sooner or later in your foolish attempt!

82

Follow These Natural Health Laws for Physical Perfection

These Natural Laws that God put in motion are the perfect laws created for your own good:

- You must eat natural foods.
- You must breathe deeply of God's air.
- You must exercise the 640 muscles of your body.
- You must give your body pure, clean water.
- You must give your body sunshine (sunbaths).
- You must not overwork your body; this leads to stress, strains, tensions and nerve depletion.
- You must keep the body clean outside and inside.
- You must live by divine intelligence and wisdom.

We are creatures of a perfect Creator. Within us is the inherent potential to become physically perfect. It is the intent of our Creator to have us have a physically perfect, healthy, happy and peaceful life!

Making positive lifestyle changes, such as daily exercise, healthy eating, eliminating stress and educating yourself about heart disease, will help lower your risk of heart disease. – Johns Hopkins Medical Letter

Enjoy Mother Nature's and God's Foods

When we are not physically perfect, we are out of harmony with the Creator's design, and therefore out of harmony with God's intent, will and law (3 John 2). In simpler words, we are, in our unhealthy living habits, opposing the will of God and Mother Earth. So, you see that to reach physical perfection, we must live correctly on all four planes: the physical, the mental, the emotional and the spiritual. By living on the physical plane correctly, we can then reach a higher mental, emotional and spiritual state.

If you eat God's and Mother Nature's foods and build a healthy, clean bloodstream, you are going to be keener mentally. The wonderful part of living by this blueprint is that we find a new calmness coming over us. You'll experience a new feeling of confidence, peace and serenity! When every cell, organ and body part is functioning perfectly, the body becomes more perfect physically, mentally, emotionally and spiritually. What complete satisfaction you will feel when you are living The Bragg Healthy Lifestyle and reaping the great rewards of a healthier, happier and more fulfilled life!

Your degree of physical perfection is the measure of your efforts in cooperating by daily partaking of proper foods, exercise, deep breathing and youthful thinking. This is your Creator's health design and intent so that you can become and remain physically healthy, youthful, active and of service, regardless of your age! Three wonderful examples that lived long lives of service: Albert Einstein, Gandhi and Albert Schweitzer.

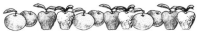

Thousands of people every year pay thousands of dollars annually for state-of-the-art testing to learn their risk for heart disease. However, experts say that fresh vegetables and a health club membership may be better buys than any lab test. People who eat a diet low in fat and cholesterol and rich in plant foods, who don't smoke, who exercise regularly, and keep their weight and blood pressure in the normal range are less likely to have a heart attack than those who don't despite any predisposition or genetic tendency toward heart disease.
– Harvard Health Letter

In quietness shall be your strength. – Isaiah 30:15

Food and Product Summary

Today, many of our foods are highly processed or refined, which robs them of essential nutrients, vitamins, minerals and enzymes. Many also contain harmful and dangerous chemicals. The research findings and experience of top nutritionists, physicians and dentists have led to the discovery that devitalized foods are a major cause of poor health, illness, cancer and premature death. The enormous increase in the last 70 years of degenerative diseases such as heart disease, arthritis and dental decay substantiate this belief. Scientific research has shown that most of these afflictions can be prevented and that others, once established, may be arrested or even reversed through nutritional methods.

Enjoy Super Health with Natural Foods

1. **RAW FOODS:** Use fresh fruits and raw vegetables, the organically grown are always best. Enjoy nutritious variety garden salads with sprouts and raw nuts and seeds.

2. **VEGETABLE and ANIMAL PROTEINS:**
   a. Legumes, lentils, brown rice, soy beans, beans.
   b. Nuts and seeds, raw and unsalted.
   c. Animal protein (if you must) – hormone free meats, liver, kidney, brain, heart, poultry, seafood. Please eat these proteins sparingly or it's best to enjoy the healthier vegetarian diet. You can bake, roast, wok or broil these proteins. Eat meat no more than 3 times a week.
   d. Dairy products – eggs (fertile, fresh), unprocessed hard cheese, goat's cheese and certified raw milk. We choose not to use dairy products. Try the healthier soy, nut (almond, etc.) and Rice Dream – the non-dairy milks.

3. **FRUITS and VEGETABLES:** Organically grown is always best – grown without the use of poisonous sprays and toxic chemical fertilizers whenever possible; ask your market to stock organic produce. Steam, bake, saute or wok veggies for as short a time as possible to retain the best nutritional content and flavor. Also enjoy fresh juices.

4. **100% WHOLE GRAIN CEREALS, BREADS and FLOURS:** They contain important B-complex vitamins, vitamin E, minerals and the important unsaturated fatty acids.

5. **COLD or EXPELLER-PRESSED VEGETABLE OILS:** Virgin olive oil, soy, sunflower, flax and sesame oils are excellent sources of healthy, essential, unsaturated fatty acids; but it's still wise to use all oils sparingly.

You are what you eat, drink, breathe, think and do! – Patricia Bragg

The Body Must Obey Your Strong, Wise Mind

Flesh is dumb! You can put anything in your stomach from coffee to hot dogs. It is not the stomach that rules the body, but your intelligent and reasoning mind! Let me close The Bragg Healthy Lifestyle Blueprint with the unequivocal statement that the properly-directed mind can inspire the body to follow this Blueprint, thereby helping the body to become closer to physical perfection.

This is God's and Our Goal for You –
Radiant, Super Health!

Blessings for Your Health, Peace, Joy, Vitality Supreme and Long-Lasting Youthfulness.

With Love,

P.S. More priceless health information follows, and we love sharing our favorite inspiring quotes with you where space allows.

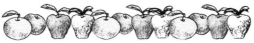

Fasting is an effective and safe method of detoxifying the body – a technique that wise men have used for centuries to heal the sick. Fast regularly and help the body heal itself and stay well!
   – James Balch, M.D., Prescription for Nutritional Healing
   "Bragg Books were my conversion to the healthy way."

85

Hippocrates, Aristotle, Galen, Paracelsus, Plato, Socrates and other great philosophers, scientists and physicians for centuries have used fasting as a method of cleansing, healing and renewing the body.

Life is to be fortified by many friendships – to love and to be loved is the greatest happiness of existence. – Sydney Smith

In nature there are neither rewards or punishments – there are consequences! – Robert Ingersoll

Avoid all self-drugging, such as aspirin and similar drugs, pain-killers, sleeping pills, tranquilizers, antihistamines, milk of magnesia, laxatives, strong cathartics and fizzing bromides. You are not qualified to prescribe drugs for yourself, and the results can be serious. – Patricia Bragg

The doctor of the future will give no medicine but will interest his patients in the care of the human frame, in diet and the cause and prevention of disease. – Thomas Edison

Avoid These Processed, Refined, Harmful Foods

Once you realize the harm caused to your body by refined, chemicalized, deficient foods, you'll want to eliminate these "killer" foods. Follow The Bragg Healthy Lifestyle for it provides the basic, essential nourishment your body needs to maintain long-lasting health.

- Refined sugar or refined sugar products such as jams, jellies, preserves, marmalades, yogurts, ice cream, sherbets, Jello, cake, candy, cookies, chewing gum, soft drinks, pies, pastries, tapioca puddings and all sugared fruit juices and fruits canned in sugar syrup. (Health stores have healthy, delicious replacements, so seek, buy and enjoy!)

- White flour products such as white bread, wheat-white bread, enriched flours, rye bread that has white flour in it, dumplings, biscuits, buns, gravy, pasta, pancakes, waffles, soda crackers, pizza, ravioli, pies, pastries, cakes, cookies, prepared and commercial puddings and ready-mix bakery products. (Health Stores have a huge variety of 100% whole grain products – delicious breads, crackers, pastas, pizzas, pastries, etc.)

- Salted foods, such as corn chips and potato chips, crackers and nuts.

- White rice and pearled barley.   • Fried and greasy foods.

- Commercial, hi-processed dry cereals made from corn, oats, etc.

- Food that contains palm and cottonseed oil. Products labeled vegetable oil . . . find out what kind before you use them.

- Peanuts and peanut butter that contains hydrogenated, hardened oils and any mold that can cause allergies.

- Margarine – full of dangerous, unnatural, trans-fatty acids.

- Saturated fats and hydrogenated oils – enemies that clog the arteries.

- Coffee, decaffeinated coffee, China black tea and all alcoholic beverages. Also all caffeinated and sugared cola and soft drinks.

- Fresh pork and pork products.   • Fried, fatty and greasy meats.

- Smoked meats, such as ham, bacon, sausage and smoked fish.

- Luncheon meats, hot dogs, salami, bologna, corned beef, pastrami and packaged meats containing dangerous sodium nitrate or nitrite.

- Dried fruits containing sulphur dioxide – a toxic preservative.

- Don't eat chickens or turkeys that have been injected with stilbestrol or fed with commercial poultry feed containing any drugs or toxins.

- Canned soups - read labels for sugar, starch, flour and preservatives.

- Food that contains benzoate of soda, salt, sugar, cream of tartar . . . and any other additives, drugs or preservatives.

- Day-old cooked vegetables, potatoes and pre-mixed, wilted salads.

- Pasteurized, filtered vinegars, distilled white, malt and synthetic vinegars – these are the dead vinegars! (We use only organic, raw, unfiltered apple cider vinegar with the "mother" as used in olden times.)

Healthy Heart Habits for Long, Vital Life

Remember, organic live foods make live people; you are what you eat, drink and do, so eat a low fat, low sugar, high fiber diet of natural whole grains and starches, sprouts, fresh salad greens, vegetables, fruits, raw seeds, nuts, pure juices and chemical-free, pure distilled water.

Earn your food with daily exercise, for regular exercise improves your health, stamina, flexibility and endurance, and helps open the cardiovascular system. Only 45 minutes a day can do miracles for your mind and body. You become revitalized with new zest for living.

We are made of tubes. To help keep them clean and open, make a mixture using ½ raw oat bran and ½ psyllium husk powder and add 1 to 3 tsp daily to juices, pep drinks, herb teas, soups, hot cereals, foods, etc. Also I take 1 cayenne capsule (40,000 HU) daily with meals.

Another way to guard against clogged tubes daily – add 2 Tbsps. soy lecithin granules, a fat emulsifier to beverages, veggies, soups, etc.

Take 50 to 100 mgs regular-released niacin (B-3) with one meal daily to help cleanse and open the cardiovascular system. Skin flushing may occur, nothing to worry about as it shows it's working! After cholesterol level reaches 180 or lower, then take 1 to 2 niacin weekly.

Your heart needs a healthy balance of nutrients, so take a natural multi vitamin-mineral food supplement with extra vitamin E (mixed tocopherols), vitamin C, magnesium orotate, selenium, zinc, beta carotene and the amino acid L-Carnitine–these are your heart's super helpers! It's also wise to take bromelain and a multi-digestive enzyme with each meal – it aids digestion, assimilation and elimination.

Many with sleep problems use melatonin or its tea for results.

Also use the amazing antioxidants pycnogenol or grape seed extract or SOD (super oxide dismutase). They help flush out dangerous free radicals that can cause havoc with your cardiovascular pipes and general health. Latest research shows extra benefits, promotes longevity, slows ageing, fights toxins, arthritis and its stiffness, swelling and pain, and helps prevent cataracts, jet lag, exhaustion and disease.

Count your blessings daily while you do your 30 to 40 minute brisk walk and exercises with these affirmations – health! strength! youth! vitality! peace! laughter! humility! understanding! forgiveness! joy! and love for eternity!– and soon all these qualities will come flooding and bouncing into your life. With blessings of super health, peace and love to you, our dear friends – our readers. – Patricia Bragg

Recommended Blood Chemistry Values

- Total Cholesterol: 180 mg/dl or less; 150 mg/dl or less is optimal
- Total Cholesterol, Childhood Years: 140 mg/dl or less
- HDL Cholesterol: Men, 50 mg/dl or more; Women, 65 mg/dl or more
- HDL Cholesterol Ratio: 3.2 or less   • Triglycerides: 100 mg/dl or less
- LDL Cholesterol: 100 mg/dl or less is optimal   • Glucose: 80-100 mg/dl

Iron Pumping Oldsters (86 to 96) Triple Their Muscle Strength in U.S. Study

WASHINGTON – Ageing nursing home residents in Boston study "pumping iron"? Elderly weightlifters tripling and quadrupling their muscle strength? Is it possible? Most people would doubt and wonder! Government experts on ageing answered those questions with a resounding "yes" with the results of this revealing and amazing study!

They turned a group of frail Boston nursing home residents, aged 86 to 96, into weightlifters to demonstrate that it's never too late to reverse age-related declines in muscle strength. The group participated in a regimen of high-intensity weight-training in a study conducted by the Agriculture Department's Human Nutrition Research Center on Ageing at Tufts University in Boston. "A high-intensity weight-training program is capable of inducing dramatic increases in muscle strength in frail men and women up to 96 years of age," reported Dr. Maria A. Fiatarone, who headed the study.

Amazing Strength Results in 8 Weeks

"The favorable response to strength training in our subjects was remarkable in light of their very advanced ages, extremely sedentary habits, multiple chronic diseases, functional disabilities and nutritional inadequacies. The elderly weight-lifters increased their muscle strength by anywhere from three-fold to four-fold in as little as eight weeks." Fiatarone said they probably were stronger at the end of the program than they had been in years!

Fiatarone and her associates emphasized the safety of such a closely supervised weight-lifting program, even among people in frail health. The average age of the 10 participants, for instance, was 90. Six had coronary heart disease; seven had arthritis; six had bone fractures resulting from osteoporosis; four had high blood pressure; and all had been physically inactive for years. Yet, no serious medical problems resulted from the program, only good outcomes!

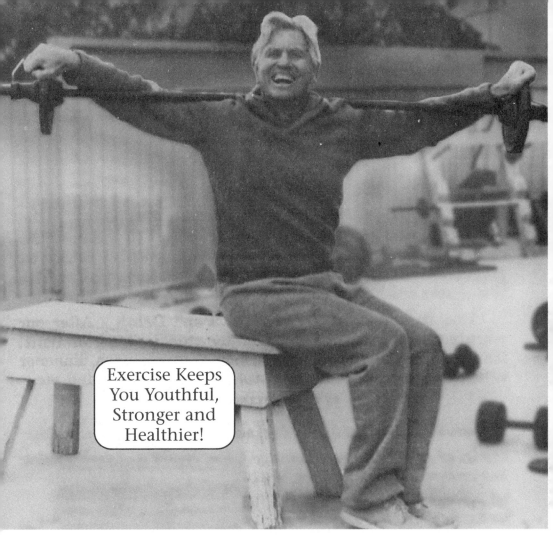

Exercise Keeps
You Youthful,
Stronger and
Healthier!

Paul C. Bragg Lifts Weights Three Times a Week

A few of the participants did report minor muscle
and joint aches, but 9 of the 10 completed the program.
One man, aged 86, felt a pulling sensation at the site of
a previous hernia incision and dropped out after 4 weeks.

The study participants, drawn from a 712 bed long-
term care facility in Boston, worked out 3 times a week.
They performed 3 sets of 8 repetitions with each leg on
a weight-lifting machine. The weights were gradually
increased from about 10 pounds initially, to about 40
pounds at the end of the eight week program.

Fiatarone said the study carries some important
implications to improve the wellness and fitness of older
people, who represent a growing proportion of the
United States population.

Muscle strength in the average adult decreases by 30% to 50% during the course of life. Experts on ageing do not know whether the decrease is an unavoidable consequence of ageing or results mainly from sedentary lifestyle and other controllable factors.

Muscle atrophy and weakness are not merely cosmetic problems in elderly people, especially the frail elderly. Researchers have linked muscle weakness with recurrent falls, a major cause of immobility and death in the American elderly population. This is causing millions of dollars yearly in staggering medical costs.

Previous studies have suggested that weight-training can be helpful in reversing age-related muscle weakness. But Fiatarone said physicians have been reluctant to recommend weight-lifting for frail elderly with multiple health problems. This new government study might be changing their minds. Also, this study shows the great importance of keeping the 640 muscles as active and fit as possible to maintain general good health.

Nature's Wonder Working Phytochemicals Help Prevent Cancer

Make sure to get your daily dose of these naturally occurring, cancer fighting biological substances, that are abundant in onions, garlic, beans, legumes, soybeans, cabbage, cauliflower, broccoli, citrus fruits, etc. The winner is tomatoes, which alone contain about 10,000 different phytochemicals!

The law, "Whatsoever a man sows that he shall also reap," is inscribed in flaming letters upon the portal of Eternity, and none can deny it, none can cheat it, none can escape it. – James Allen

Nutrition directly affects growth, development, reproduction, well-being of an individual's physical and mental condition. Health depends upon nutrition more than on any other single factor. – Dr. Wm. H. Sebrell, Jr.

Alternative Health Therapies And Massage Techniques

Explore these wonderful natural methods of healing your body. Then choose the technique best for you:

Acupuncture/Acupressure – Acupuncture directs and rechannels body energy by inserting hair-thin needles (use only disposable needles) at specific points on the body. It's used for pain, backaches, migraines and general body disfunction. Used in Asia for centuries, acupuncture is safe, virtually painless and has no side effects. Acupressure is based on the same principles and uses finger pressure and massage rather than needles.

Chiropractic – Daniel David Palmer founded chiropractic in 1885 in Davenport, Iowa. There are now 16 schools in the U.S., from which graduates are joining Health Practitioners in all the modern nations of the world to share healing techniques. Chiropractic is the largest healing profession and benefits millions. Treatment involves soft tissue, spinal and body adjustment to free the nervous system of interferences with normal body function. Its concern is the functional integrity of the musculoskeletal system. In addition to manual methods, chiropractors use physical therapy modalities, exercise, health and nutritional guidance.

F. Mathius Alexander Technique – Lessons intended to end improper use of neuromuscular system and bring body posture back into balance. Eliminates psycho-physical interferences, helps release long-held tension, and aids in re-establishing muscle tone.

Feldenkrais Method – Founded by Dr. Moshe Feldenkrais in the late 1940s. Lessons lead to improved posture and help create ease and efficiency of movement. A great stress removal method.

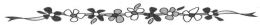

Who is strong? He that can conquer his bad habits. – Ben Franklin

Caring hands have healing lifeforce energy . . . babies love and thrive with daily massages and cuddles. Family pets love soothing, healing touches. Everyone benefits from healing massages and treatments! – Patricia Bragg

Homeopathy – Dr. Samuel Hahnemann developed homeopathy in the 1800s. Patients are treated with minute amounts of substances similar to those that cause a particular disease to trigger the body's own defenses. The homeopathic principle is *like cures like*. This safe and nontoxic remedy is the #1 alternative therapy in Europe and Britain because it is inexpensive, seldom has any side effects, and gets amazing, fast results.

Naturopathy – Brought to America by Dr. Benedict Lust, M.D., this treatment uses diet, herbs, homeopathy, fasting, exercise, hydrotherapy, manipulation and sunlight. (Dr. Paul Bragg was a graduate of Dr. Lust's first Naturopathic School in the U.S.) Practitioners work with your body to restore health naturally. They reject surgery and drugs except as a last resort.

Osteopathy – The first School of Osteopathy was founded in 1892 by Dr. Andrew Taylor Still, M.D. There are now 15 such colleges in the U.S. Treatment involves soft tissue, spinal and body adjustments that free the nervous system from interferences that can cause illness. Healing by adjustment also includes good nutrition, physical therapies, proper breathing and good posture. Dr. Still's premise was that structure and function of the human body are interdependent; if the body structure is altered or abnormal, function is altered and illness results.

Reflexology or Zone Therapy – Founded by Eunice Ingham, author of "The Story The Feet Can Tell," whose health career was inspired by a Bragg Health Crusade when she was 17. Reflexology helps the body by removing crystalline deposits from meridians (nerve endings) of the feet through deep pressure massage. A form of Reflexology has its early origins in China and is known to have been practiced by Kenyan natives and North American Indian tribes for centuries. Reflexology helps to activate the body's natural flow of healthy energy by dislodging the collected deposits.

Reiki – A Japanese form of massage that means "Universal Life Energy." Reiki helps the body to detoxify, then rebalance and heal itself. Discovered in the ancient Sutra manuscripts by Dr. Mikso Usui in 1822.

Rolfing – A technique developed by Ida Rolf in the 1930s in the U.S., variously called structural processing, postural release or structural dynamics. It is based on the concept that distortions of normal function of organs and skeletal muscles occur throughout life and are accentuated by the effects of gravity on the body. Rolfing helps the individual to achieve balance and improved body posture. Methods involve the use of stretching, deep tissue massage and relaxation techniques to loosen old injuries and break bad movement and posture patterns, which can cause long-term body stress.

Tragering – Founded by Dr. Milton Trager M.D., who was inspired at age 18 by Paul C. Bragg to become a doctor. It is an experimental learning method that involves gentle shaking and rocking, suggesting a greater letting go, releasing tensions and lengthening of muscles for more body health. Tragering can do miraculous healing where needed in the muscles and the entire body.

Water Therapy – For a great shower, apply almond, avocado, sesame or olive oil to skin, then alternate hot and cold water and massage needed areas while under spray. Garden hose massage is great in summer. Tub baths are wonderful: apply oil and massage. For muscle aches, add 1 cup apple cider vinegar or Epsom salts.

93

Dry Skin Brushing (brush lightly) is wonderful for circulation, toning and healing. For variety use a loofah sponge for massaging in the shower and tub.

Massage – Aromatic – It works two ways: the essence (smell) helps the patient relax as does the massage itself, while the massage is used to help absorption of essential natural oils used for centuries to treat numerous complaints. For example, Tiger Balm, echinacea and arnica help relieve muscle aches. Avoid creams and lotions with mineral oil because it clogs the skin's pores. Almond, avocado and olive oils are good and the most popular. There are over 40 aromatics to use derived from herbs and other botanicals. (Pure rosemary oil, 6 drops to 6 ounces of almond oil, is a favorite.)

When health is absent, wisdom cannot reveal itself, strength cannot be exerted, wealth is useless and reason is powerless. – Herophiles, 300 B.C.

Massage – Self – Paul C. Bragg often said, "You can be your own best massage therapist, even if you have only one good hand." Near-miraculous improvements have been achieved by victims of accidents or strokes in bringing life back to afflicted parts of their own bodies by self-massage and even vibrators. Treatments can be day or night, almost continual. Also, self-massage can help achieve relaxation at day's end. Families and friends can learn and exchange massages; it's a wonderful sharing experience. Remember, babies also love and thrive with daily massages – start from birth. Your family pets also love the soothing, healing touch of massage.

Massage – Shiatsu – Japanese form of massage that applies pressure from the fingers, hands, elbows and even knees along the same points as acupuncture. Used in Asia for centuries to relieve pain, common ills, muscle stress and to aid lymphatic circulation.

Massage – Sports – An important support system for professional and amateur athletes. Sports massage: improves circulation and mobility to injured tissue, enables athletes to recover more rapidly from myofascial injury, reduces muscle soreness and chronic strain patterns. Soft tissues are freed of trigger points and adhesions, thus contributing to improvement of peak neuro-muscular functioning and athletic performance.

Massage – Swedish – One of the oldest and most-used massage techniques. It's deep body massage that soothes, promotes circulation and is also a great way to loosen and relax muscles before and after exercise.

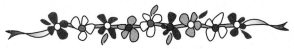

Author's Comment: My father and I have personally sampled many of these techniques. It's estimated that by the year 2000 U.S. Health Care costs will reach over $2 trillion. It's more important than ever that we be responsible for our own health. This includes seeking holistic health practitioners who are dedicated to keeping us well by inspiring us to practice prevention! These Alternative Healing Therapies are also popular and getting results – color, aroma, music, biofeedback, Tai Chi, yoga, etc. Explore them and be open to improving your earthly temple for a healthy, happy, longer life.

Seek and find the best for your body, mind and soul. – Patricia Bragg.

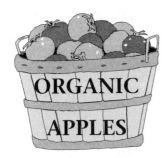

Food For Thought

Fruit bears the closest relation to light. The sun pours a continuous flood of light into the fruits, and they furnish the best potion of food a human being requires for the sustenance of mind and body. – Alcott

The purest food is fruit, next vegetables, then cereals. All pure poets have abstained almost entirely from animal food. Especially a minister should eat less meat, when he has to write and give a sermon. They say the less meat, the better the sermon. – Amos Bronson Alcott

There is much false economy: those who are too poor to have seasonable fruits and vegetables, will yet have pie and pickles all the year. They cannot afford oranges, yet can afford tea and coffee daily. – Health Calendar

The men who kept alive the flame of wisdom, learning and piety in the Middle Ages were mainly vegetarians. – Sir William Axon

95

If families could be induced to substitute the healthy organic apple, sound, ripe and luscious, in place of white sugar, white flour pies, cakes, candies and other sweets with which children are too often stuffed, doctors' bills would diminish sufficiently enough in a single year to lay up a stock of this delicious fruit for a season's use.

Through the law of cause and effect we choose our destiny through life. Moreover, we are our own prophets, for we constantly project our future state by the seeds we plant in the present. – Cheryl Canfield

DO MORE TO MAKE LIFE SUCCESSFUL

Do more than preach, practice.
Do more than think, ponder.
Do more than sympathize, empathize.
Do more than scold, set an example.
Do more than criticize, praise.
Do more than dream, make it a reality!

– Rev. Paul Osumi, Honolulu, Hawaii

These freshly squeezed organic vegetable and fruit juices are important to The Bragg Healthy Lifestyle. It's not wise to drink beverages with your main meals, as it dilutes the digestive juices. But it's great during the day to have a glass of freshly squeezed orange, grapefruit, vegetable juice, Bragg Vinegar Drink, herb tea or try a hot cup of Bragg Liquid Aminos Broth (½ to 1 tsp Bragg Liquid Aminos in cup of hot distilled water) – these are all ideal pick-me-up beverages.

Bragg Apple Cider Vinegar Cocktail – Mix 1-2 tsp. equally of Bragg Organic ACV and (optional) raw honey or pure maple syrup in distilled water. Take 1 glass upon arising, an hour before lunch and dinner.

Delicious Hot Cider Drink – Add a few cinnamon sticks and cloves to hot distilled water and let steep for 20 mins. Before drinking add 2 tsps Bragg Raw Organic Apple Cider Vinegar and raw honey equally.

Bragg Favorite Juice Cocktail – This drink consists of all raw vegetables (please remember organic is best) which we prepare in our vegetable juicer: carrots, celery, beets, cabbage, watercress and parsley. The great purifier, garlic we enjoy but it's optional.

Bragg Favorite Healthy "Pep" Drink – After our morning stretch and exercises we often enjoy this instead of fruit. It's also delicious and powerfully nutritious as a meal anytime: lunch, dinner or take along in a thermos to work, school, the gym, or to the park or hiking, etc.

Bragg Healthy Pep Drink

Prepare the following in blender, add 1 ice cube if desired colder: *Choice of: freshly squeezed orange juice, grapefruit or tangelo; carrot and greens juice; unsweetened pineapple juice; or 1½ cups distilled water with:*

½ tsp raw wheat germ	¼ tsp vitamin C powder
⅓ tsp flaxseed oil, optional	¼ tsp nutritional yeast flakes
¼ tsp green powder (barley, etc.)	1 to 2 bananas, ripe
½ tsp raw oat bran	1 tsp raw honey, optional
½ tsp psyllium husk powder	1 tsp soy protein powder
½ tsp lecithin granules	1 tsp raw sunflower seeds

Optional: 4 apricots (sun dried, unsulphured). Soak in jar overnight in distilled water or unsweetened pineapple juice. We soak enough to last for several days. Keep refrigerated. In summer, you can add fresh fruit in season: peaches, strawberries, berries, apricots, etc. instead of the banana. In winter, add apples, kiwi, oranges, pears or persimmons or try sugar-free, frozen organic fruits. Serves 1 to 2.

Patricia's Delicious Health Popcorn

Use freshly popped popcorn (I prefer air popped). If desired, use olive, soy, sesame or flax seed oil or melted salt-free butter. Pour the oil over popcorn and then add several sprays of Bragg Liquid Aminos and Bragg ACV. Sprinkle with nutritional yeast large flakes. Add pinch of Italian or French herbs, cayenne pepper, mustard powder or fresh crushed garlic to the oil mixture. Delicious served instead of breads!

Bragg Lentil & Brown Rice Casserole

14 oz pkg lentils, uncooked
4 carrots, chopped
3 celery stalks, chopped
2 onions, chopped
3 quarts distilled water

4 garlic cloves, chopped
1 cup brown rice, uncooked
1 tsp Bragg Liquid Aminos
¼ tsp Italian herbs (oregano, basil, etc.)
2 tsp olive oil (virgin - cold-pressed is best)

Wash & drain lentils and rice. Place grains in large stainless steel pot. Add water. Bring to boil, reduce heat & simmer for 30 minutes. Add vegetables & seasonings & cook on low heat until done. Just before serving, you may add fresh or canned tomatoes. For a delicious garnish add parsley & nutritional yeast large flakes. Add more water in cooking the grains for a delicious soup or stew. Serves 4 to 6.

Bragg Raw Vegetable Garden Salad

2 stalks celery, chopped
1 bell pepper & seeds, diced
½ cucumber, chopped
1 carrot, grated
1 raw beet, grated
1 cup green cabbage, sliced

½ cup red cabbage, chopped
½ cup alfalfa or sunflower sprouts
2 spring onions & tops, chopped
1 turnip, grated
1 avocado (ripe)
3 tomatoes, medium size

97

For variety add raw zucchini, sugar peas, mushrooms, broccoli, cauliflower. Dice avocado & tomato and serve on side as a dressing. Chop, slice or grate vegetables fine to medium for variety in size. Mix vegetables thoroughly & serve on a bed of lettuce, spinach, watercress or chopped cabbage. Serve choice of fresh squeezed lemon, orange or dressing separately. Chill salad plates before serving. Always eat salad first before serving hot dishes. Serves 3 to 5.

Bragg Vinaigrette Health Dressing

½ cup Bragg Apple Cider Vinegar
2 tsps raw honey
⅓ tsp Bragg Liquid Aminos
1 to 2 cloves garlic, minced
⅓ cup virgin olive oil, or blend with flax, soy or sesame oils
1 Tbsp fresh herbs, minced or pinch Italian or French dry herbs

Blend ingredients in blender or jar. Refrigerate in covered jar.

For delicious herbal vinegar: in quart jar add ⅓ cup tightly packed, crushed fresh sweet basil, tarragon, dill, oregano, or any fresh herbs desired, combined or singly. (If *dried* herbs, use 1 to 2 tsp. herbs.) Now cover to top with Bragg Organic Raw Apple Cider Vinegar and store 2 weeks in warm place, strain and refrigerate.

Honey – Celery Seed Vinaigrette

¼ tsp dry mustard
¼ tsp Bragg Liquid Aminos
¼ tsp paprika
3 Tbsp raw honey

1 cup Bragg Apple Cider Vinegar
½ cup virgin olive oil
1 medium onion, minced
⅓ tsp celery seed

Blend ingredients in blender or jar. Refrigerate in covered jar.

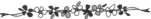

Healthy, organic foods have a wonderful abundance of potential life energy.

Take Time for 12 Things

1. Take time to **Work** –
   it is the price of success.
2. Take time to **Think** –
   it is the source of power.
3. Take time to **Play** –
   it is the secret of youth.
4. Take time to **Read** –
   it is the foundation of knowledge.
5. Take time to **Worship** –
   it is the highway of reverence and
   washes the dust of earth from our eyes.
6. Take time to **Help and Enjoy Friends** –
   it is the source of happiness.
7. Take time to **Love** –
   it is the one sacrament of life.
8. Take time to **Dream** –
   it hitches the soul to the stars.
9. Take time to **Laugh** –
   it is the singing that helps life's loads.
10. Take time for **Beauty** –
    it is everywhere in nature.
11. Take time for **Health** –
    it is the true wealth and treasure of life.
12. Take time to **Plan** –
    it is the secret of being able to have time
    for the first 11 things.

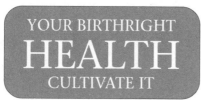

YOUR BIRTHRIGHT
HEALTH
CULTIVATE IT

Have an

Apple

Healthy Day!

Teach me Thy way O Lord, and Lead me in
Thy plain path. – Psalms 27:11

Exercise and Eat for Health

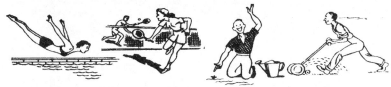

The Bragg Healthy Lifestyle
For a Lifetime of Super Health

In a broad sense, "The Bragg Healthy Lifestyle for the Total Person" is a combination of physical, mental, emotional, social and spiritual components. The ability of the individual to function effectively in his environment depends on how smoothly these components function as a whole. Of all the qualities that comprise an integrated personality, a totally healthy, fit body is one of the most desirable . . . so start working today to achieve your health goals!

A person may be said to be totally physically fit if he functions as a total personality with efficiency and without pain or discomfort of any kind. This is to have a Painless, Tireless, Ageless body, possessing sufficient muscular strength and endurance to maintain a healthy posture and successfully carry on the duties imposed by life and the environment, to meet emergencies satisfactorily and have enough energy for recreation and social obligations after the "work day" has ended. It is to meet the requirements for his environment through possessing the resilience to recover rapidly from fatigue, tension, stress and strain of daily living without the aid of stimulants, drugs or alcohol, and enjoy natural recharging sleep at night and awaken fit and alert in the morning for the challenges of the fresh new day ahead.

Keeping the body totally healthy and fit is not a job for the uninformed or the careless person. It requires an understanding of the body and of a healthy lifestyle and then following that lifestyle for a long, happy life. The result of "The Bragg Healthy Lifestyle" is to wake up the possibilities within you, rejuvenate your body, mind and soul to total, balanced health. It's within your reach, so don't procrastinate, start today! Our hearts go out to touch your heart and mind with nourishing, caring love for your total health!

With Love, Patricia Bragg and Paul C. Bragg

Dear friend, I wish above all things that thou may prosper and be in health even as the soul prospers. – 3 John 2

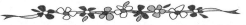

Nature and its beauty is the signature of God.

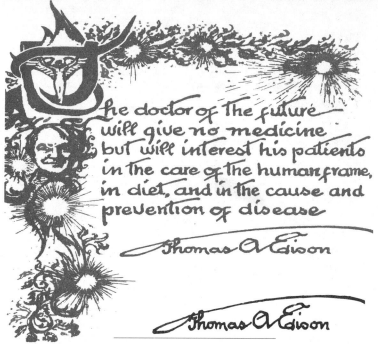

The doctor of the future will give no medicine but will interest his patients in the care of the human frame, in diet, and in the cause and prevention of disease

Thomas A Edison

Thomas A Edison

Healthy Fiber for Super Health

- EAT BERRIES, surprisingly good sources of fiber.

- KEEP BEANS HANDY, probably the best fiber sources. Cook dried beans and freeze in portions. Use canned beans for faster meals.

- INSTEAD OF ICEBERG LETTUCE, choose deep green lettuces, romaine, bib, butter, etc., spinach or cabbage for variety salads.

- LOOK FOR "100% WHOLE WHEAT" or whole grain breads. A dark color isn't proof; check labels, compare fibers, grains, etc.

- WHOLE GRAIN CEREALS. Hot , also cold granolas with sliced fruit.

- GO FOR BROWN RICE. It's better for you and so delicious.

- EAT THE SKINS of potatoes and other fruits and vegetables.

- LOOK FOR CRACKERS with at least 2 grams of fiber per ounce.

- SERVE HUMMUS, made from chickpeas, instead of sour-cream dips.

- USE WHOLE-WHEAT FLOUR for baking breads, muffins, pastries, pancakes, waffles and for variety try other whole grain flours.

- DON'T UNDERESTIMATE CORN, including popcorn, corn tortillas.

- ADD OAT BRAN, WHEAT BRAN AND WHEATGERM to baked goods, cookies, etc.; whole grain cereals, casseroles, loafs, etc.

- SNACK ON SUN-DRIED FRUIT, such as apricots, dates, prunes, raisins, etc., which are concentrated sources of nutrients and fiber.

- INSTEAD OF DRINKING JUICE, eat the fruit, orange, grapefruit, etc.; and vegetables , tomato, carrot, etc. – UC Berkeley Wellness Letter

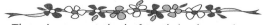

There is a great deal of truth in the saying that man becomes what he eats. – Gandhi

Foods and Allergies

Every known food may cause some allergic reaction at times. Thus the foods used in "elimination" diets may cause allergic reactions in some individuals and a few are listed among the "Most Common Food Allergies." Since the incidence of reaction to these foods is generally low, they are widely used in making test diets. By keeping your own food journal you will soon know your "problem" foods that must be eliminated from your diet.

After eating some particular type of food and especially if it happens each time you eat that food, your body has a reaction, the chances are you may have an allergy. Here are some of the allergic reactions and they can happen very quickly! If you wheeze, sneeze, develop a stuffy nose, nasal drip or mucus, dark circles or waterbags under your eyes, headaches, feel light-headed or dizzy, heart beats faster, stomach and chest pains, diarrhea, extreme thirst, break out in a rash or have a swelling of the tissues, (ankles, feet, hands or stomach bloating, etc.) either externally or internally.

If you know what your allergy is, you are lucky; if you don't, you had better find out as fast as possible and eliminate all irritating foods from your diet. To re-evaluate your daily life, as a guide to your future start a daily journal (8½ x 11 notebook) of foods eaten and your reactions, moods, energy levels, weight, elimination and sleep patterns. Soon you will discover the foods and situations causing your problems. By charting your activities you will be amazed at the swings following eating certain foods. Paul C. Bragg faithfully kept a journal for over 70 years.

If you are hypersensitive to certain foods, you must reject them from your diet! There are hundreds of allergies and of course it is impossible here to take up each one. Many who suffer from this unpleasant affliction have allergies to wheat, milk or eggs, while some persons are allergic to all grains. Your journal will help you discover and accurately pinpoint the foods and situations causing your problems. Start today!

Most Common Food Allergies

- CEREALS: *Buckwheat, Corn, Oats, Rye, Wheat*
- MILK: *Butter, Cheese, Cottage Cheese, Ice Cream, Milk, etc.*
- EGGS: *Cakes, Custards, Dressings, Mayonnaise, Noodles*
- FISH: *Shellfish, Crabs, Lobster, Shrimp, Shadroe*
- MEATS: *Bacon, Chicken, Pork, Sausage, Veal*
- FRUITS: *Citrus Fruits, Melons, Strawberries*
- VEGETABLES: *Brussels Sprouts, Cauliflower, Celery, Eggplant, Legumes, Onions, Potatoes, Spinach, Tomatoes*
- NUTS: *Peanuts, Pecans, Walnuts*
- MISCELLANEOUS: *Chocolate, China Tea, Cocoa, Coffee, Palm and Cottonseed Oils, MSG, Salt, Spices*

We don't endorse white vinegar or dead vinegars for human use – internally nor externally! But it seems well-suited for a variety of household and workshop chores. White vinegar is an effective and inexpensive household cleaner, deodorizer and disinfectant; which replaces commercial household cleaners that are full of chemicals and additives harmful to Mother Nature and you. But please remember: use only the healthiest raw, organic unfiltered apple cider vinegar (with the "mother") for all human consumption and for your skin and hair.

VINEGAR USES FOR KITCHEN CLEANING

• **Appliances and Countertops:** clean and disinfect with vinegar-dampened sponge or cloth.

• **Greasy Areas:** mix ¼ cup vinegar with 2 cups hot water and add 1 to 2 dashes of biodegradable liquid soap. (Keep mixture in handy, labeled spray bottle.)

• **Sponges and Dish Rags:** disinfect and deodorize by soaking overnight in 1 quart hot water with ¼ cup vinegar.

102

• **Chopping and Bread Boards:** wipe down with full-strength white vinegar to disinfect; or sprinkle with baking soda before spraying with vinegar, wait 30 minutes before wiping clean, then rinse with water.

• **Pots and Pans:** clean and polish with paste of baking soda and vinegar. Remove stubborn, stuck-on food with a 50/50 vinegar-water soak.

• **Glass and China:** stop spotting by mixing ½ cup vinegar in dishwater, or by placing 1 cup vinegar on bottom rack of electric dishwasher before starting wash.

• **Drains and Pipes:** keep fresh-smelling and free-flowing with ½ cup of baking soda followed by ½ cup of vinegar. Cover drain opening with plate for an hour or longer before flushing through with cold water.

• **Garbage Disposals:** keep clean by grinding up frozen vinegar ice cubes (80/20 vinegar-water solution to make cleansing ice cubes).

Of all the gifts that a wise providence grants us to make life fuller and happier – friendship is the most beautiful. – Epicurus

---

The secret of longevity largely is eating intelligently. – Gayelord Hauser

VINEGAR USES FOR THE BATHROOM

• **Chrome and Stainless Steel:** straight vinegar will disinfect and polish fixtures; apply with sponge, then buff with soft cloth.

• **Toilet Bowl:** use ½ cup straight vinegar, let stand an hour or more and flush. For bad stains, follow vinegar with sprinkle of biodegradable cleanser; after 2 hours brush and flush. If stains persist use Clorox bleach (½ cup) overnight.

• **Sink, Tub and Shower:** spray with 80/20 vinegar-water mixture, leave 5 minutes, then scrub and rinse.

• **Shower Curtains:** put through washer rinse cycle with 1 to 2 cups vinegar. Spray with 50/50 vinegar-water solution to help prevent mold.

• **Garbage Pails:** disinfect with a warm water and vinegar solution. Let set for an hour or overnight.

VINEGAR USES FOR THE LAUNDRY ROOM

• **Washer Tub and Hoses:** remove soap accumulations by running machine for full cycle with pint of vinegar.

• **New Clothes, Linens, etc:** to remove manufacturing chemicals and new smell odors, add 1 to 2 cups vinegar to first wash before using.

• **Perspiration Odor and Stained Clothes:** soak overnight in ¼ cup vinegar and enough water to cover or soak in washer or pan, then wash in morning.

• **Clothes Final Rinse Cycle:** to help remove static and lint add ½ cup vinegar.

• **To Soften and Disinfect Fabric, Clothes etc:** add ¼ cup vinegar to most loads.

• **Fruit and Grass Stains:** dab with straight vinegar within 24 hours to safely remove most stains and spots.

• **Musky Smells:** to remove odor and freshen clean cotton clothes just sprinkle with vinegar and press.

• **Steam Iron Plate:** to eliminate mineral deposits, fill iron reservoir with straight vinegar and allow to steam on rag, then fill with plain water and turn upside down and drain.

• **Scorched Fabric:** gently rub with vinegar, then wipe with clean, white cloth.

Never underestimate the power of a kind word or deed.

VINEGAR USES FOR FLOORS, WALLS & FURNITURE

• **Windows:** spray 50/50 vinegar-water mixture, then wipe clean with squeegee. (Great for eye glasses.)

• **Floors:** sponge mop with 1 cup of vinegar in a bucket of warm water. Also removes dull residue left by most commercial cleaners.

• **Carpets:** light stains are extracted using a mix of 2 Tbsps. salt and ½ cup vinegar; rub paste into carpet and allow to dry before vacuuming.

• **Furniture:** remove cloudy look & brighten by rubbing with a mixture of 1 Tbsps. vinegar in a quart of warm water, then buff with soft cloth. Remove white rings from tables with a mixture of equal parts vinegar and olive oil.

• **Vinyl Surfaces:** wipe down with 2 Tbsps. liquid soap and ½ cup vinegar before rinsing with water and drying.

• **Toys:** Clean and disinfect with a light spray of vinegar (50/50 vinegar-water solution) and brush or wipe clean.

• **Air Freshener:** mask kitchen odors by simmering a pot of water with ½ cup vinegar.

(104)

VINEGAR USES FOR OUTSIDE

• **Car & Car Windows:** keep frost-free with coating solution of 50/50 vinegar to water. Also, dissolve old decals and chewing gum with straight vinegar.

• **Paint Brushes:** soften by soaking in boiling vinegar; also, remember that vinegar absorbs paint odors!

• **Ants:** spray equal parts vinegar and water on areas where an ant invasion might or has occurred; vinegar works as a non-toxic "pesticide."

• **Fresh-Cut Flowers:** preserve by adding 2 Tbsps. vinegar to quart of warm water in flower vase.

• **Unwanted Grass & Weeds:** pour on straight vinegar.

God will not change the condition of men,
until they change what is in themselves. – Koran

There is no such thing as too many friends, just as there
is never too much happiness! – Jean de La Bruyere

Happiness is a rainbow in your heart – a real health sparkler!
– Patricia Bragg

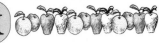

Index

105

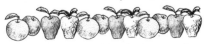

*We are recharged and blessed by each one of you reading our
loving, health – inspirational teachings. Thank you!* – Patricia Bragg

*It's never too late to begin getting into shape, but it
does take daily perseverance.* – Thomas K. Cureton

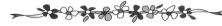

Love is not a matter of counting the years –
it's making the years count. – William Smith

Always do what is right – despite any public opinions.

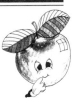

**HAVE AN
APPLE
HEALTHY LIFE!**

*"I conceive that a knowledge of books is the basis on which
all other knowledge rests."* – George Washington, 1st U.S. President

What sunshine is to flowers, smiles are to humanity. – Joseph Addison

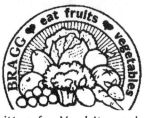

FROM THE AUTHORS

GO ORGANIC

This book was written for You! It can be your passport to a healthy, long, vital life. We in the Alternative Health Therapies join hands in one common objective – promoting a high standard of health for everyone. Healthy nutrition points the way – which is Mother Nature and God's Way. This book teaches you how to work with them, not against them. Health d octors, therapists nurses, teachers and caregivers are becoming more dedicated than ever to keep their patients healthy and fit. This book was written to speed the spread of this tremendous message of living a healthy lifestyle close to Mother Nature and God.

Statements in this book are scientific health findings, known facts of physiology, biological therapeutics. Paul C. Bragg practiced the natural methods of living for over 80 years with highly beneficial results, knowing that they were safe and of great value. His daughter Patricia Bragg worked with him to carry on the Bragg Health Crusades.

Paul C. Bragg and daughter Patricia express their opinions solely as Public Health Educators and Health Crusaders. They offer no cure for disease. Only the body has the ability to cure a person. Experts may disagree with some of the statements made in this book. However, such statements are considered to be factual, based upon the long-time health experience of pioneer Paul C. Bragg and Patricia Bragg. If you suspect you have a medical problem, please seek alternative health professionals to help you make the healthiest, wisest and best-informed choices.

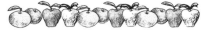

Bragg Blessings to You, Our Treasured Friends

From the Bragg home to yours we share our health knowledge – years of living close to God and Mother Nature. What joys of fruitful, radiant living this produces – this my Father and I want to share with you and your loved ones. With Love and Blessings for Health, Peace and Happiness.

May you prosper in good health as well as your soul prospers. – 3 John 2

To maintain good health, normal weight and increase the good life of radiant health, joy and happiness, the body must be exercised properly (stretching, walking, jogging, running, biking, swimming, deep breathing, good posture, etc.) and nourished wisely with natural foods. – Paul C. Bragg

Send for Free Health Bulletins

Let Patricia Bragg send you, your relatives and friends the latest discoveries on Health, Nutrition, Exercise and Longevity. These are sent free periodically. All donations and gifts are tax deductible and appreciated for our spreading the gospel of health to everyone, including schools, churches, prisons and institutions, etc. Also, your donations will help fund our planned Health Retreats which are needed now more than ever! For more information please see page vi up front.

With Blessings of Health and Thanks,

Patricia

Please print or type addresses clearly . . .

BRAGG HEALTH CRUSADES, Box 7, Santa Barbara, CA 93102

●
_____
Name
                                    (   ) _____
_____
Address   Phone

_____
City   State   Zip Code

●
_____
Name
                                    (   ) _____
_____
Address   Phone

_____
City   State   Zip Code

●
_____
Name
                                    (   ) _____
_____
Address   Phone

_____
City   State   Zip Code

●
_____
Name
                                    (   ) _____
_____
Address   Phone

_____
City   State   Zip Code

●
_____
Name
                                    (   ) _____
_____
Address   Phone

_____
City   State   Zip Code

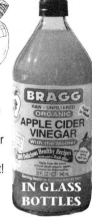

– Make copies of order form to use – if unavailable in your area –

BRAGG "HOW-TO, SELF-HEALTH" BOOKS

Authored by America's First Family of Health
Live Longer – Healthier – Stronger Self-Improvement Library

Qty.	Bragg Book Titles ORDER FORM Health Science ISBN 0-87790	Price	$ Total
____	**Apple Cider Vinegar — Miracle Health System**	6.95	.
____	**The Bragg Healthy Lifestyle - Vital Living to 120** (formerly Toxicless Diet)	7.95	.
____	**Super Power Breathing for Super Energy – High Health & Longevity**	7.95	.
____	**Miracle of Fasting** (Bragg Bible of Health for physical rejuvenation & longevity)	8.95	.
____	**Water – The Shocking Truth** (learn safest water to drink & why)	7.95	.
____	**Nature's Healing System to Improve Eyesight** in 90 days (foods, exercises, etc.)	7.95	.
____	**Bragg's Complete Gourmet Recipes** for Vital Health – 448 pages	8.95	.
____	**Bragg Health & Fitness Manual** – Triathlon Manual – Swim-Bike-Run – for All Ages		
	A Must for Athletes, Triathletes & would-be-athletes – 600 pages	16.95	.
____	**Build Powerful Nerve Force** (reduce stress, fear, anger, worry)	7.95	.
____	**Keep Your Heart & Cardiovascular System Healthy & Fit** at Any Age	7.95	.
____	**Nature's Way to Reduce** (lose 10 pounds in 10 days)	6.95	.
____	**Hair and Your Health**, Nature's Way to Beautiful Hair (easy-to-do method)	7.95	.
____	**Sauerkraut & Cabbage Recipes** Raw, Salt-Free (make your own – it's so healthy)	2.95	.
____	**Healthy, Strong Feet** – "Best Complete Foot Progam" – Dr. Scholl	7.95	.
____	**Fitness/Spine Motion** – For a More Flexible, Pain-free Back	3.95	.
____	**Nature's Way to Health** (simple method for long, healthy life to 120)	6.95	.

Total Copies Prices subject to change without notice.

TOTAL BOOKS $.

USA Shipping Please add $2 for first book, $1 for each additional book. USA retail book orders over $35 add $5 only.

CA residents add sales tax .

Shipping & Handling .

Canada & Foreign orders add $2 per book. (USA Funds Only)

TOTAL ENCLOSED $ (USA Funds Only) .

Please Specify: ☐ Money Order ☐ Cash ☐ Check

Charge To: ☐ Visa ☐ Master Card ☐ Discover   Month Year

Credit Card Number: ___ ___ ___ ___   Card Expires: ___ | ___

Signature: _____

CREDIT CARD ORDERS ONLY
CALL (800) 446-1990
OR FAX (805) 968-1001

Business office calls **(805) 968-1020.** We accept MasterCard Discover or VISA phone orders. Please prepare your order using this order form. It will speed your call and serve as your order record. Hours: 9 am to 4 pm Pacific Time, Monday thru Thursday.
Visit our Web Site: http://www.bragg.com & e-mail: bragg@bragg.com

Mail to: **HEALTH SCIENCE, Box 7, Santa Barbara, CA 93102 USA**
Please Print or Type – Be sure to give street & house number to facilitate delivery.

BOF- 807

Name

Address   Apt. No.

City   State
Phone (   )   ● Zip

Bragg Books available most Health & Book Stores – Nationwide

BRAGG ALL NATURAL LIQUID AMINOS

Delicious, Healthy Seasoning Alternative to Tamari & Soy Sauce

BRAGG LIQUID AMINOS — Nutrition you need...taste you will love...a family favorite for over 85 years. A delicious source of nutritious life-renewing protein from soybeans only. Add to or spray over casseroles, soups, sauces, gravies, potatoes, popcorn, and vegetables. An ideal "pick-me-up" broth at work, home or the gym. Gourmet health replacement for Tamari and Soy Sauce. Start today and add more Amino Acids to your daily diet for healthy living — the easy BRAGG LIQUID AMINOS Way!

SPRAY or DASH brings NEW TASTE DELIGHTS! PROVEN & ENJOYED BY MILLIONS.

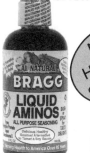

Now in Handy 6 oz Spray Bottle

Spray or Dash of Bragg Aminos Brings New Taste Delights to Season:
- Salads
- Dressings
- Soups
- Veggies
- Tofu
- Rice/Beans
- Tempeh
- Stir-frys
- Wok foods
- Gravies
- Sauces
- Meats
- Poultry
- Fish
- Popcorn
- Casseroles & Potatoes
- Macrobiotics

Pure Soybeans and Pure Water Only
- No Added Sodium
- No Coloring Agents
- No Preservatives
- Not Fermented
- No Chemicals
- No Additives

BRAGG LIQUID AMINOS

SIZE	PRICE	USA SHIPPING & HANDLING	AMT	$ TOTAL
6 oz.	$ 2.98 ea.	Please add $3 for 1st 3 bottles – $1.25 each additional bottle.		•
6 oz.	$ 68.54 Case/24	S/H Cost by Time Zone: CA $5. PST/MST $7. CST $9. EST $11.		•
16 oz.	$ 3.95 ea.	Please add $3 for 1st bottle – $1.25 each additional bottle.		•
16 oz.	$ 43.45 Case/12	S/H Cost by Time Zone: CA $6. PST/MST $7. CST $10. EST $11.		•
32 oz.	$ 6.45 ea.	Please add $4 for 1st bottle – $1.50 each additional bottle.		•
32 oz.	$ 70.95 Case/12	S/H Cost by Time Zone: CA $8. PST/MST $11. CST $16. EST $19.		•

Bragg Liquid Aminos is a food and not taxable

Foreign orders, please inquire on postage

Please Specify: ☐ Check ☐ Money Order ☐ Cash

Charge To: ☐ Visa ☐ MasterCard ☐ Discover

Total Aminos	$	•
Shipping & Handling		•
Total Enclosed (USA Funds Only)	$	•

Credit Card Number: _ _ _ _ — _ _ _ _ — _ _ _ _ — _ _ _ _   Card Expires: Month | Year

MasterCard *VISA* DISCOVER   **Signature:** _____

CREDIT CARD ORDERS ONLY
CALL **(800) 446-1990**
OR FAX **(805) 968-1001**

Business office calls (805) 968-1020. We accept MasterCard Discover or VISA phone orders. Please prepare your order using this order form. It will speed your call and serve as your order record. Hours: 9 am to 4 pm Pacific Time, Monday thru Thursday.
Visit our Web Site: http://www.bragg.com & e-mail: bragg@bragg.com

Mail to: HEALTH SCIENCE, Box 7, Santa Barbara, CA 93102 USA

Please Print or Type – Be sure to give street & house number to facilitate delivery.

A-BOF- 807

• Name

• Address   Apt. No.

• City   State

Phone ( )   • Zip

Bragg Aminos – Taste You Love, Nutrition You Need!
Available Health Stores - Nationwide

Bragg Organic Raw Apple Cider Vinegar
With the Mother . . . Nature's Delicious, Healthy Miracle

**HAVE AN
APPLE
HEALTHY DAY!**

– IF ? –

Your Favorite Health Store
doesn't carry
Bragg Raw Organic Vinegar
Ask them to Contact their
Health Distributor to stock it!
Or they can Call
Bragg at 1-800-446–1990

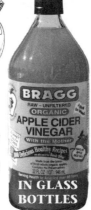

**IN GLASS
BOTTLES**

INTERNAL BENEFITS:
- Rich Miracle Enzymes & Potassium
- Natural Antibiotic & Germ Fighter
- Helps Control & Normalize Weight
- Improves Digestion & Assimilation
- Helps Fight Arthritis & Stiffness
- Relieves Sore & Dry Throats
- Helps Remove Toxins & Sludge

EXTERNAL BENEFITS:
- Helps Promote Youthful, Healthy Body
- Helps Promote & Maintain Healthy Skin
- Soothes Sunburn, Shingles & Bites
- Helps Prevent Dandruff & Itchy Scalp
- Soothes Aching Joints & Muscles

BRAGG ORGANIC APPLE CIDER VINEGAR

SIZE	PRICE	USA SHIPPING & HANDLING	AMT	$ TOTAL
16 oz.	$ 2.19 ea.	Please add $3 for 1st bottle and $1.50 each additional bottle		
16 oz.	$24.09 Case/12	S/H Cost by Time Zone: CA $7. PST/MST $8. CST $12. EST $14.		
32 oz.	$ 3.79 ea.	Please add $4 for 1st bottle and $2.00 each additional bottle.		
32 oz.	$41.69 Case/12	S/H Cost by Time Zone: CA $10. PST/MST $14. CST $20. EST $24.		

Bragg Vinegar is a food and not taxable

Foreign orders, please inquire on postage.

Please Specify: ☐ Check ☐ Money Order ☐ Cash

Charge To: ☐ Visa ☐ MasterCard ☐ Discover

Credit Card
Number:

Total Vinegar $	
Shipping & Handling	
Total Enclosed $ (USA Funds Only)	

Month Year
Card Expires: ____ | ____

Signature: _____

CREDIT CARD ORDERS ONLY
CALL **(800) 446-1990**
OR FAX **(805) 968-1001**

Business office calls (805) 968-1020. We accept MasterCard Discover or VISA phone orders. Please prepare your order using this order form. It will speed your call and serve as your order record. Hours: 9 am to 4 pm Pacific Time, Monday thru Thursday.
Visit our Web Site: http://www.bragg.com & e-mail: bragg@bragg.com

Mail to: **HEALTH SCIENCE, Box 7, Santa Barbara, CA 93102 USA**

Please Print or Type – Be sure to give street & house number to facilitate delivery.

V-BOF-807

Name

Address   Apt. No.

City   State

Phone ( )   Zip

Bragg Apple Cider Vinegar – Taste You Love, Health You Need!
Available Health Stores - Nationwide

BRAGG ALL NATURAL LIQUID AMINOS

Delicious, Healthy Seasoning Alternative to Tamari & Soy Sauce

BRAGG LIQUID AMINOS — Nutrition you need...taste you will love...a family favorite for over 85 years. A delicious source of nutritious life-renewing protein from soybeans only. Add to or spray over casseroles, soups, sauces, gravies, potatoes, popcorn, and vegetables. An ideal "pick-me-up" broth at work, home or the gym. Gourmet health replacement for Tamari and Soy Sauce. Start today and add more Amino Acids to your daily diet for healthy living — the easy BRAGG LIQUID AMINOS Way!

SPRAY or DASH brings NEW TASTE DELIGHTS! PROVEN & ENJOYED BY MILLIONS.

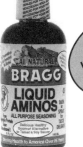

Now in Handy 6 oz Spray Bottle

Spray or Dash of Bragg Aminos Brings New Taste Delights to Season:

- Salads
- Dressings
- Soups
- Veggies
- Tofu
- Rice/Beans
- Tempeh
- Stir-frys
- Wok foods
- Gravies
- Sauces
- Meats
- Poultry
- Fish
- Popcorn
- Casseroles & Potatoes • Macrobiotics

Pure Soybeans and Pure Water Only

- No Added Sodium
- No Coloring Agents
- No Preservatives
- Not Fermented
- No Chemicals
- No Additives

BRAGG LIQUID AMINOS

SIZE	PRICE	USA SHIPPING & HANDLING	AMT	$ TOTAL
6 oz.	$ 2.98 ea.	Please add $3 for 1st 3 bottles – $1.25 each additional bottle.		•
6 oz.	$68.54 Case/24	S/H Cost by Time Zone: CA $5. PST/MST $7. CST $9. EST $11.		•
16 oz.	$ 3.95 ea.	Please add $3 for 1st bottle – $1.25 each additional bottle.		•
16 oz.	$43.45 Case/12	S/H Cost by Time Zone: CA $6. PST/MST $7. CST $10. EST $11.		•
32 oz.	$ 6.45 ea.	Please add $4 for 1st bottle – $1.50 each additional bottle.		•
32 oz.	$70.95 Case/12	S/H Cost by Time Zone: CA $8. PST/MST $11. CST $16. EST $19.		•

Bragg Liquid Aminos is a food and not taxable

Foreign orders, please inquire on postage

Please Specify: ☐ Check ☐ Money Order ☐ Cash

Charge To: ☐ Visa ☐ MasterCard ☐ Discover

Total Aminos $	•
Shipping & Handling	•
Total Enclosed $ (USA Funds Only)	•

Credit Card Number: _ _ _ _ _ _ _ _ _ _ _ _ _ _ _ _   Card Expires:___|___   Month | Year

MasterCard VISA DISCOVER   **Signature:** _____

CREDIT CARD ORDERS ONLY
CALL **(800) 446-1990**
OR FAX **(805) 968-1001**

Business office calls (805) 968-1020. We accept MasterCard Discover or VISA phone orders. Please prepare your order using this order form. It will speed your call and serve as your order record. Hours: 9 am to 4 pm Pacific Time, Monday thru Thursday.
Visit our Web Site: http://www.bragg.com & e-mail: bragg@bragg.com

Mail to: **HEALTH SCIENCE, Box 7, Santa Barbara, CA 93102 USA**

Please Print or Type – Be sure to give street & house number to facilitate delivery.

A-BOF- 807

•
Name

•
Address   Apt. No.

•   •
City   State
Phone (   )   • Zip

Bragg Aminos – Taste You Love, Nutrition You Need!
Available Health Stores - Nationwide

BRAGG "HOW-TO, SELF-HEALTH" BOOKS

Authored by America's First Family of Health
Live Longer – Healthier – Stronger Self-Improvement Library

Qty.	Bragg Book Titles ORDER FORM Health Science ISBN 0-87790	Price	$ Total
_____	**Apple Cider Vinegar – Miracle Health System**	6.95	.
_____	**The Bragg Healthy Lifestyle - Vital Living to 120** (formerly Toxicless Diet)	7.95	.
_____	**Super Power Breathing for Super Energy – High Health & Longevity**	7.95	.
_____	**Miracle of Fasting** (Bragg Bible of Health for physical rejuvenation & longevity)	8.95	.
_____	**Water – The Shocking Truth** (learn safest water to drink & why)	7.95	.
_____	**Nature's Healing System to Improve Eyesight** in 90 days (foods, exercises, etc.)	7.95	.
_____	**Bragg's Complete Gourmet Recipes** for Vital Health – 448 pages	8.95	.
_____	**Bragg Health & Fitness Manual** – Triathlon Manual – Swim-Bike-Run – for All Ages		.
	A Must for Athletes, Triathletes & would-be-athletes – 600 pages	16.95	.
_____	**Build Powerful Nerve Force** (reduce stress, fear, anger, worry)	7.95	.
_____	**Keep Your Heart & Cardiovascular System Healthy & Fit** at Any Age	7.95	.
_____	**Nature's Way to Reduce** (lose 10 pounds in 10 days)	6.95	.
_____	**Hair and Your Health**, Nature's Way to Beautiful Hair (easy-to-do method)	7.95	.
_____	**Sauerkraut & Cabbage Recipes** Raw, Salt-Free (make your own – it's so healthy)	2.95	.
_____	**Healthy, Strong Feet** – "Best Complete Foot Progam" – Dr. Scholl	7.95	.
_____	**Fitness/Spine Motion** – For a More Flexible, Pain-free Back	3.95	.
_____	**Nature's Way to Health** (simple method for long, healthy life to 120)	6.95	.

Total	
☐ **Copies** Prices subject to change without notice.	**TOTAL BOOKS** $.
USA Shipping 〉 Please add $2 for first book, $1 for each additional book. USA retail book orders over $35 add $5 only.	**CA residents add sales tax** .
	Shipping & Handling .
Canada & Foreign orders add $2 per book. (USA Funds Only)	**TOTAL ENCLOSED** $. (USA Funds Only)

Please Specify: ☐ Money Order ☐ Cash ☐ Check

Charge To: ☐ Visa ☐ Master Card ☐ Discover   Month   Year

Credit Card Number: __ __ __ __ — __ __ __ __ — __ __ __ __ — __ __ __ __   Card Expires: ___|___

MasterCard VISA DISCOVER   **Signature:** _____

Business office calls (805) 968-1020. We accept MasterCard Discover or VISA phone orders. Please prepare your order using this order form. It will speed your call and serve as your order record. Hours: 9 am to 4 pm Pacific Time, Monday thru Thursday.
Visit our Web Site: http://www.bragg.com & e-mail: bragg@bragg.com

Mail to: **HEALTH SCIENCE, Box 7, Santa Barbara, CA 93102 USA**

Please Print or Type – Be sure to give street & house number to facilitate delivery.
BOF- 807

•
Name

•
Address   Apt. No.

•   •
City   State
Phone (   )   • Zip

Bragg Books available most Health & Book Stores – Nationwide

Send for Free Health Bulletins

Let Patricia Bragg send you, your relatives and friends the latest discoveries on Health, Nutrition, Exercise and Longevity. These are sent free periodically. All donations and gifts are tax deductible and appreciated for our spreading the gospel of health to everyone, including schools, churches, prisons and institutions, etc. Also, your donations will help fund our planned Health Retreats which are needed now more than ever! For more information please see page vi up front.

With Blessings of Health and Thanks,

Patricia

Please print or type addresses clearly . . .

BRAGG HEALTH CRUSADES, Box 7, Santa Barbara, CA 93102

●

Name _____

Address _____ ( ) _____ Phone

City _____ State _____ Zip Code _____

●

Name _____

Address _____ ( ) _____ Phone

City _____ State _____ Zip Code _____

●

Name _____

Address _____ ( ) _____ Phone

City _____ State _____ Zip Code _____

●

Name _____

Address _____ ( ) _____ Phone

City _____ State _____ Zip Code _____

●

Name _____

Address _____ ( ) _____ Phone

City _____ State _____ Zip Code _____

PAUL C. BRAGG N.D., Ph.D.

Life Extension Specialist • World Health Crusader
Lecturer and Advisor to Olympic Athletes, Royalty and Stars
Originator of Health Food Stores – Now Worldwide

For almost a Century, Living Proof that his
"Health and Fitness Way of Life" Works Wonders!

Paul C. Bragg is the Father of the Health Movement in America. This dynamic Crusader for worldwide health and fitness is responsible for more *firsts* in the history of the Health Movement than any other individual.

Bragg's amazing pioneering achievements the world now enjoys:

- Bragg originated, named and opened the first Health Food Store in America.
- Bragg Health Crusades pioneered the first Health Lectures across America. He inspired followers to open health stores across America and also worldwide.
- Bragg introduced pineapple juice and tomato juice to the American public.
- He was the first to introduce and distribute honey nationwide.
- He introduced Juice Therapy in America by importing the first hand-juicers.
- Bragg pioneered Radio Health Programs from Hollywood three times daily.
- Paul and Patricia pioneered a Health TV show from Hollywood to spread *Health and Happiness* . . . the name of the show! It included exercises, health recipes, visual demonstrations and guest appearances by famous, health-minded people.
- He opened the first health restaurants and the first health spas in America.
- He created the first health foods and products and made them available nationwide: herb teas, health beverages, seven-grain cereals and crackers, health cosmetics, health candies, calcium, vitamins and mineral supplements, wheat germ, digestive enzymes from papaya, herbs and kelp seasonings, and amino acids from soybeans. Bragg inspired others to follow (Schiff, Shaklee, Twin Labs, Herbalife, etc.) and now thousands of health items are available worldwide.

Crippled by TB as a teenager, Bragg developed his own eating, breathing and exercising program to rebuild his body into an ageless, tireless, pain-free citadel of glowing, radiant health. He excelled in running, swimming, biking, progressive weight training and mountain climbing. He made an early pledge to God, in return for his renewed health, to spend the rest of his life showing others the road to health. He honored his pledge! Bragg's health pioneering made a big difference worldwide.

A living legend and beloved counselor to millions, Bragg was the inspiration and personal health and fitness advisor to top Olympic Stars from 4-time swimming Gold Medalist Murray Rose to 3-time track Gold Medalist Betty Cuthbert of Australia, his relative (pole-vaulting Gold Medalist) Don Bragg and countless others. Jack LaLanne, the original TV Fitness King , says, *"Bragg saved my life at age 15 when I attended the Bragg Crusades in Oakland, California."* From the earliest days, Bragg advised the greatest Hollywood Stars and giants of American Business. Del E. Webb, JC Penney, Dr. Scholl and Conrad Hilton are just a few who he inspired to long, successful, healthy active lives!

Dr. Bragg changed the lives of millions worldwide in all walks of life with the Bragg Health Crusades, Books, Tapes, Radio and TV appearances.

BRAGG HEALTH CRUSADES, Box 7, SANTA BARBARA, CA 93102 USA

PATRICIA BRAGG N.D., Ph.D.

Angel of Health and Healing

Author, Lecturer, Nutritionist, Health Educator & Fitness Advisor to World Leaders, Hollywood Stars, Singers, Dancers & Athletes

Daughter of the world renowned health authority, Paul C. Bragg, Patricia has won international fame on her own in this field. She conducts Health and Fitness Seminars for Women's, Men's, Youth and Church Groups throughout the world . . . and promotes Bragg "How-To, Self-Health" Books in Lectures, on Radio and Television Talk Shows throughout the English-speaking world. Consultants to Presidents and Royalty, to the Stars of Stage, Screen and TV and to Champion Athletes, Patricia and her father are Co-Authors of the Bragg Health Library of Instructive, Inspiring Books that promote a longer, vital, healthier lifestyle.

Patricia herself is the symbol of health, perpetual youth and super energy. She is a living and sparkling example of her and her father's healthy lifestyle precepts and this she loves sharing worldwide.

A fifth-generation Californian on her mother's side, Patricia was reared by The Bragg Natural Health Method from infancy. In school, she not only excelled in athletics, but also won honors for her studies and her counseling. She is an accomplished musician and dancer . . . as well as tennis player and mountain climber . . . and the youngest woman ever to be granted a U.S. Patent. Patricia is a popular gifted Health Teacher and a dynamic, in-demand talk show guest where she spreads the simple, easy-to-follow Bragg Healthy Lifestyle for everyone of all ages.

Man's body is his vehicle through life, his earthly temple . . . and the creator wants us filled with joy & health for a long fruitful life. The Bragg Crusades of Health and Fitness (3 John 2) has carried her around the world over 10 times – spreading physical, spiritual, emotional, mental health and joy. Health is our birthright and Patricia teaches how to prevent the destruction of our health from man-made wrong habits of living.

Patricia's been a Health Consultant to American Presidents and British Royalty, to Betty Cuthbert, Australia's "Golden Girl," who holds 16 world records and four Olympic gold medals in women's track and to New Zealand's Olympic Track and Triathlete Star, Allison Roe. Among those who come to her for advice are some of Hollywood's top Stars from Clint Eastwood to the ever-youthful singing group, The Beach Boys and their families, Singing Stars of the Metropolitan Opera and top Ballet Stars. Patricia's message is of worldwide appeal to people of all ages, nationalities and walks-of-life. Those who follow the Bragg Healthy Lifestyle and attend the Bragg Crusades worldwide are living testimonials . . . like ageless, super athlete, Jack LaLanne, who at age 15 went from sickness to Total Health!

Patricia Bragg inspires you to Renew, Rejuvenate and Revitalize your life with "The Bragg Healthy Lifestyle" Seminars and Lectures worldwide. These life-changing events are where millions have benefitted with a longer, healthier life! Patricia loves to share with your community, organization, church groups, etc. Also, she is a perfect radio and TV talk show guest to spread the message of super healthy lifestyle living.

For Radio interview requests and info write or call (800) 446-1990
BRAGG HEALTH CRUSADES, BOX 7, SANTA BARBARA, CA 93102, USA